Pregnant!
What Can I Do?

Pregnant!
What Can I Do?

A Guide for Teenagers

by Tania Heller, M.D.

McFarland & Company, Inc., Publishers
Jefferson, North Carolina, and London

Library of Congress Cataloguing-in-Publication Data

Heller, Tania, 1958–
   Pregnant! what can I do? : a guide for teenagers / by Tania
Heller
     p.   cm.
   Includes bibliographical references and index.
   ISBN 0-7864-1169-4 (softcover : 60# alkaline paper) ∞
   1. Teenage mothers—United States. 2. Teenage pregnancy—
United States. I. Title.
HQ759.4.H45   2002
306.874'3—dc21   2001007177

British Library cataloguing data are available

Manufactured in the United States of America

Cover photograph by Marty McGee

McFarland & Company, Inc., Publishers
  Box 611, Jefferson, North Carolina 28640
   www.mcfarlandpub.com

To my husband Sam and my children Daniel and Ariel,
who teach me so much about parenting every day

Contents

Preface

I still remember as if it were yesterday, the day one of my classmates in tenth grade disappeared from high school with no good-byes. Only years later did I discover that she had been pregnant and had been taken out of school in shame – to parent the baby, or have an abortion? I may never know. She left no forwarding address. Those were the only options spoken about in those days, certainly amongst high school girls and boys. The idea of a third option never entered my mind. Although adoption was usually more common a generation ago it was often done secretly and almost never as an "open adoption." There was usually no contact between the birth-parents, adoptive parents and child.

As a pediatrician I've treated children and young adults for almost 20 years. During that time I've seen many teenagers with unwanted pregnancies, and not much has changed. The teenage pregnancy and abortion rates were (and still are) too high, and perhaps because of shame and embarrassment, not much is spoken about a third option, namely adoption.

I wrote this book to present, without judgment, all three options available to pregnant teenagers. In this book I also strongly emphasize the prevention aspect; i.e., preventing an unwanted pregnancy with its consequences. Last but not least, I provide an easy-to-read guide to the decision-making process and where to go for help, and discuss the importance of taking care of yourself physically and mentally during pregnancy.

I am grateful to my parents, Izzy and Zelda Heller, and my grandmother Fay Dektor, for their love and support.

Thank you to Heather Boonstra and Rachel Jones at the Alan Guttmacher Institute, Caren Hiser at "Adoptions Together," and psychiatrist and author Dr E. James Lieberman. A special thanks also to my patients, and to all the pregnant teenagers who were willing to share their life stories with me. I have changed their names in order to protect their privacy.

Introduction

Adolescence is a time when you are faced with important decisions about your education, career, sexual relationships and possibly marriage. Your decisions are influenced by your family and friends, as well as by social and economic circumstances. The choices you make now will strongly affect the rest of your life, including your educational achievement and employment opportunities.

When is one ready for parenthood? Any parent will tell you that true commitment and strength are required to bring up a child. Most adolescents, by virtue of the emotional and physical changes that they are going through and struggles they must face, are not ready to make that commitment. It is certainly not an ideal time to be taking on the full responsibility of another human being.

That having been said, in the United States, just under a million adolescent women become pregnant each year. About three quarters of teenage pregnancies are unintended, and more than a quarter end in abortion. Only a small percentage of pregnant teenagers opt for adoption. Although the 1990s saw a definite decline in teenage pregnancy rates and birth rates (*Family Planning Perspectives*, Vol. 32, no. 5, Sept./Oct., 2000, and National Center for Health Statistics) the United States teen pregnancy rate is still one of the highest in the developed world.

Most American teenagers have sex for the first time between the ages of 15 and 17. More than a third of ninth graders and two thirds of 12th graders have had sexual intercourse (A.A.P. "Pediatrics" Nov., 1999). Several factors contribute to the high rate of teenage sexual activity and teenage pregnancy. Personal factors, such as low self-esteem, family factors including lack of discipline and overly permissive parenting, societal factors, such as lack of education (including contraceptive education), and our permissive society, all play a role.

There is good news too. Between 1990 and 1997, the teenage pregnancy and birth rates fell significantly. The decline in teenage pregnancy is thought by some to be due to increased abstinence or increased contraceptive use, by others to a fear of HIV, and by yet others, to a combination of the above.

Discussion of premarital sex, pregnancy and abortion engenders strong personal feelings in most individuals. In this book I try to present the facts in an unbiased and nonjudgmental manner, respecting the reader's personal beliefs and legal rights.

What's the problem?

When looking at the major problems our society faces, certainly teenage pregnancy, abortion and sexually transmitted disease rank high on the list. What is the scope of the problem and why do we spend so much time looking at these issues?

Every year almost one million teenagers become pregnant in the United States. In fact the teenage pregnancy and teenage birth rates in the U.S. are higher than in any other industrialized country in the world. Adolescent pregnancy carries with it a large number of problems for the teenager and her partner, their families and society.

More than three quarters of the teenage pregnancies in the U.S. each year are unplanned and unintended. It is sad to note that whereas the birth rate for married women is about ten times the abortion rate, in unmarried women the birth and abortion rates are nearly equal. Induced abortion is the most commonly performed surgical procedure in the United States.

There is some good news. The teenage pregnancy rate dropped significantly between 1988 and 1996 and in that same time period the teen abortion rate dropped by 33 percent. However the numbers are still too high. Although studies indicate that most younger teenage girls are not sexually active, by 17, more than half have had sexual intercourse, and a sexually active teenager who does not use contraceptives has a 90 percent chance of becoming pregnant within a year.

Younger teenagers having sex for the first time usually use a condom. When sexually experienced teenagers use contraception, the method most commonly used is the oral contraceptive pill (44 percent), followed by the condom. A smaller number rely on other methods, including the injectable, the withdrawal method, the diaphragm, the sponge and the implant. However, many teenagers practice contraception sporadically or not at all. (Refer to Chapter 9 for more information about contraception.)

Besides unplanned pregnancy, teenagers face the threat of sexually transmitted diseases. Teenage women are at higher risk than older women of acquiring such diseases. Every year three million teenagers—about one in four sexually experienced teenagers—contracts at least one sexually transmitted disease. These include gonorrhea, genital herpes, chlamydia, human papillomavirus, syphilis and HIV amongst others. There is a very high incidence of chlamydia in sexually active teenagers—as high as about 10 to 30 percent in some settings. Complications of chlamydia and gonorrhea include pelvic inflammatory disease, infertility and ectopic pregnancy. Teenage women have a higher hospitalization rate than older women for acute pelvic inflammatory disease. It is important to be aware that women with chlamydia may have no symptoms at all, but still develop serious complications, so you must be tested for this infection if you are sexually active. Other sexually transmitted infections, too, are very prevalent amongst teenagers. One quarter of all new HIV infections occur among 13- to 21-year-olds (Office of National AIDS policy, 1996).

The cost of treating the complications of sexually transmitted diseases is very high. Approximately four to five billion dollars are spent each year (Lappa & Moscicki, Dec., 1997). Although there are some costs incurred in preventing sexually transmitted diseases, they are not nearly as high as treating them.

The cost to society and taxpayers of teenage pregnancy in general is also high. The estimated cost of births to young women who became mothers when they were 15 to 17, instead of 20 to 21 years old, is at least $6.9 billion.

Early sexual activity is associated in some cases with other problem behaviors, such as not performing as well at school, using illegal drugs, and having a history of criminal involvement.

Problems of Teenage Pregnancies

A teenage pregnancy is often a high-risk pregnancy. Having a baby is one of the most significant events in a person's life. Having one during adolescence is much more complicated and potentially hazardous than having a baby as an adult. The risks to both mother and baby are higher.

For a number of reasons, including lack of health insurance, pregnant teenagers are less likely and less able than older women to obtain early and regular prenatal care (*Family Planning Perspectives*, Vol. 32, no.5). This can result in pregnancy-related complications not being identified and treated. Other factors, such as a small pelvic size in the mother due to incomplete bone growth, and poor nutrition, can also affect outcome. The babies of teenage mothers are more likely to be born prematurely and at a lower birth weight. Both of these factors increase the risk of other problems in the child, including respiratory problems.

Pregnancy, birth and infant complications are higher if there is a history of tobacco, alcohol or drug use in the mother. In addition other associated circumstances, such as maternal depression, lack of support and inadequate finances, all play a role.

The situation becomes very serious and complicated if a teenager becomes pregnant through sexual assault or incest (sexual abuse committed by a family member). Although help is available, it is sad to note that most incest cases are never reported, often due to fear or lack of trust.

Some of the factors associated with early sexual activity and teenage pregnancy:

• Family structure: According to the National Campaign to Prevent Teen Pregnancy, teenagers from intact two-parent families are less likely to give birth in their teens than girls in other family situations.

• Teenage girls whose mothers gave birth in their teens have sex and get pregnant earlier than girls whose mothers had their first child at 20 years or later.

• Teenage girls whose mothers did not graduate from high school have a higher chance of having sex and giving birth in their teens than girls whose mothers finished high school.

Most teenage pregnancies are unintended. Some are intended, but the reasons may not reflect mature judgment. A young woman might believe that a pregnancy would bring her closer to her partner, or she might want a baby to give her the love she does not receive elsewhere.

Teenage mothers who carry their pregnancies to term may raise their babies on their own or with the help of their parents, family members or the father. Only about one in five unmarried teenage mothers ever receives financial support from the teenage father. Even if a teenage mother marries the father and has his support, she still needs to understand the limitations on her freedom that motherhood imposes. Teenage mothers are less likely to finish high school or attend college (only a third receive a high school diploma); therefore, they are less likely to find a good job, and more likely to end up on welfare (nearly 80 percent of unmarried teen mothers end up on welfare). Their relationships with friends often become strained, because of their lack of time and energy to socialize. Teenage mothers often have a second and even a third baby, which can make it more difficult for them to finish school or earn a good living. A third of teen mothers 16 and younger have a second child within two years. This puts the family at higher risk of poverty. Poverty is one of the causes as well as a consequence of teenage pregnancy. For a number of reasons teenage mothers are often unable to provide the kind of environment that babies and very young children need for optimal development.

Although many of the negative consequences for teenage mothers are due to their poor situations prior to pregnancy, having a baby at an early age can make matters worse. The divorce rate in teenage marriage is very high. Studies on children brought up in single homes, without a father present, indicate that children fare best in the presence of a two-parent loving family. When compared with children in similar situations who live with two parents, children who grow up with one parent are more likely to drop out of high school, become teen mothers, and be out of a job.

However, this is not always the case, and in Chapter 4 I discuss situations in which women took control and made the best of difficult situations, with good outcomes.

Problems with Health Care for Teenagers

A survey by the Kaiser Family Foundation found that while more than half the teenagers they interviewed said they had some information about sex and birth control, many said it did not include enough detail about how to use or where to obtain contraceptives. Many pregnant teenagers don't know where to turn for help.

A problem for male teenagers is that the United States is sorely lacking in reproductive health care services for men. Women have opportunities to discuss sexuality and their sexual health at their routine gynecological visit, or if they present to a clinic for contraception or pregnancy. Young men are often only examined at routine school or sports physicals, when many of these important issues are not discussed.

Young men are not routinely asked about sexual relationships or concerns relating to sexuality, nor are they routinely screened for sexually transmitted diseases, unless they present with a specific concern. Both males and females should be responsible for their sexuality and their choices, and so I believe that all teenagers need to be offered comprehensive health services, including preventive services, and counseling when needed. Men should feel comfortable about discussing these issues with their doctors.

Your physician (primary care physician or obstetrician) or counselor should be able to give you a list of available resources and clinics in your area that deal with sexually transmitted diseases and pregnancy-related issues for yourself and your partner. You can also call your local Planned Parenthood Affiliate for further information. In Appendix B of this book you will also find a list of resources.

2

How could it happen to me?

Finding out that you are pregnant creates all sorts of emotions. You may feel happy, scared, shocked and sad, sometimes almost all at once. You may want to deny the fact that you could be pregnant. Some of the thoughts you may have are: what will my parents do? what will my friends say? what will happen to my schooling? where will I find money? should I run away? what will this do to my looks? will I get fat?

Unmarried pregnant teenagers face many decisions: whether to give birth or terminate the pregnancy; if the former, whether to raise the baby or place the baby for adoption. At the same time they face all the decisions about school, work and relationships that other teenagers face.

Too often I hear young men and women tell me they never believed this could happen to them. You will read about Amy and Rami later in the book. They used no contraception and were still surprised when Amy became pregnant. It reminds me of when I was young and had just earned my driver's license. I knew one shouldn't drive too fast and I knew people who had been involved in car accidents, but I couldn't imagine that could ever happen to me. As one gets older one's perspective certainly changes. Yes, accidents can happen to you if you drive too fast, and you too can become pregnant if you have sex and don't use contraception.

Sheila was 19 years old, with a 23-year-old not-too-steady boyfriend. She was a second year college student, in the prime of her life, when she found out that she was pregnant. They had been using condoms with foam. Sheila was concerned about the side effects of the pill, although she had not really discussed this with her doctor.

The two of them had gone to a party until late one night. That night was the one and only night they did not use a condom. Looking back, Sheila doesn't know if they forgot, or if they were too tired. Either way, soon after that she missed a period, and could hardly bring herself to the store to buy a home pregnancy test, she was shaking so much. When she saw the positive result, she felt as if her life had been shattered. She could never have imagined that something like this could happen to her. "Your whole life changes. All your freedom is gone. Only faith could get me through this." Sheila had to make a lot of changes during her pregnancy. She transferred to a community college away from her friends, so that she could live at home, and she took on extra jobs to pay the bills. Sheila told me that she soon realized who her true friends were. Only a few stood by her as she gave up her social life, and she sadly lost contact with her boyfriend after he received the news of her pregnancy.

Andrea was only 14 years old—a ninth grader—when she became pregnant. "I was stupid. I knew it would happen. Okay, I kind of wanted it to happen in a way. We think it will be easy. It's not! It changes your whole life." Andrea wasn't feeling well. When she missed her period, she did a urine home pregnancy test and wasn't surprised to learn that she was pregnant. It was only days later that the full impact hit her. "My parents were very mad. They treated me so badly. My boyfriend was happy in the beginning, but when he heard about my plan to give the baby up for adoption, he became angry and we never got along again. He wanted to bring the baby up with the help of his mom. He didn't even want me in the picture!" Andrea also lived with her parents throughout her pregnancy, but felt most supported by her grandpa and some of her friends.

Andrea has since given her baby up for adoption, and has a semiopen arrangement. She keeps in touch with the baby and the adoptive family through letter writing and photographs. How is Andrea doing? "I feel pretty good, knowing I did the right thing for my baby. I still have pangs of sadness sometimes though."

Possible Reactions to an Unplanned Pregnancy

Pregnant teenagers experience all sorts of emotions throughout pregnancy. They may be sad, angry, hopeful and scared—sometimes all at the same time. Here are just a few common reactions:

DENIAL

Denial is a common reaction to a difficult or very sad situation. Some women go into a stage of denial about their pregnancies. This is a way of helping them cope with a situation too difficult to face, until they are ready to deal with it. When a woman is in this stage it is very difficult to get the help for her to move on.

Rebecca, age 16, was in denial about her situation for weeks. She found it difficult to talk to anyone about her situation. When reality hit her, she withdrew from her friends and her family. She neglected herself and ate irregularly. Rebecca became ill before she finally agreed to go for help.

SADNESS AND DEPRESSION

Depression can be expressed in many different ways. Some women feel deep sadness, anxiety and poor concentration. They may lose interest in activities they used to enjoy, may neglect themselves, eat poorly, and withdraw from family and friends. In the case of an unwanted pregnancy, they may be mourning the loss of their innocence, the loss of their childhood, and the loss of the chance of an intact happy family.

Maria, a 16-year-old high school student, became pregnant only two months after she began dating Brad. Although they were sexually active, she was afraid to discuss going on the pill with either her parents or her physician. Brad thought condoms reduced sensation, so they practiced the withdrawal method.

When she first developed some nausea, and found she was starting to go to the bathroom more often, she thought she had a urinary tract infection. She didn't think she had really missed a period, although the last one had been much lighter than usual. At no time did pregnancy cross her mind.

Maria went to her pediatrician to get tested and treated for the urinary tract infection, but instead found that her pregnancy test was positive. She was devastated. Her doctor and the nurses spent time with her, counseling her and talking about her options, but Maria couldn't hear much at all. She didn't want to tell her parents at the time. She couldn't tell her boyfriend, because she didn't know where he was. All Maria could do was take down the name of an obstetrician-gynecologist, and promise she would go for an appointment soon.

Maria went home and went straight to bed. All sorts of bad thoughts filled her mind. She didn't have anyone to confide in. How would she go to school? Who would help her look after her baby? She had read scary stories about abortions. Should she leave home? If so, where could she go?

She decided to skip school the next day and told her mother she had a fever.

The phone rang the next Saturday afternoon. Her best friend invited her to come along to a movie. When Maria hesitated, then declined, sobbing, Sharon, who knew her very well, decided to come right over. The friends trusted each other, so Maria opened up, and found that once she had confided in someone her relief was tremendous. She felt like a huge weight had been lifted off her shoulders. She now had strength to do something, rather than lie in bed feeling sorry for herself. That night she spoke to her mother, and on Monday, she picked up the crumpled note from her doctor, and made the first call to the obstetrician.

GUILT

Guilt is a deep feeling of having done something wrong. You have probably all had some experience with guilt. You may be putting all the blame on yourself for this pregnancy. It might be worth looking at the question: why did I get pregnant when I did?

• You may not have been able to get to the doctor's office for a prescription for the pill or the diaphragm.
• You may not have had the money to buy contraception at the time.
• You may have been "caught up in the moment" and not used contraception that one time.
• You may have been using a method of contraception that was not very reliable, such as withdrawal.

Sometimes there are more complex reasons for why you became pregnant when you did.

• Were you coerced into having sex?
• Did you subconsciously want to get pregnant?
• Were you testing your relationship?
• Did you believe a pregnancy would bring you closer together?

Ava Torre-Bueno, a licensed clinical social worker, says in her book, *Peace After Abortion*, that it is often unconscious motivation that leads women not to use birth control and to have an unwanted pregnancy. So it may not be necessary to blame yourself.

It is important to understand those motivations, though, so that you can look to a better future and prevent this from happening again.

SHAME

Some women with whom I have spoken have said that they were dealing mostly with shame. This emotion led them to hide their pregnancies as long as possible and prevented them from speaking to family, friends or counselors early on. Some of them went on to have abortions.

Many pregnant teenagers are afraid to talk to their parents or even their boyfriends. Others are anxious about revealing their pregnancies to their employers, friends or teachers. They may not know who to turn to.

There is help at hand! See a doctor (and counselor if necessary) as soon as possible. Don't put your life and possibly the baby's life in jeopardy. This is a time to do a lot of thinking, and a lot of talking, to your parents or other trusted family members, friends, counselor or doctor. Learn about all your options, but don't delay, because the longer you wait the fewer options you will have.

3

Taking control

"O Wind, If Winter comes, can Spring be far behind?"
— Percy Bysshe Shelley (1792–1822)
"Ode to the West Wind" (1819)

Even though it may feel as if you have lost all control, this is not so. You do have control with respect to decision making now. You can decide whether you will raise this baby, or opt for adoption or abortion. If you decide to raise your baby, you will decide to parent with or without a partner. Many things factor into this decision-making process and it isn't easy, but you can start taking control now. Believe in yourself, but also get help in making your decision. Each option has advantages and disadvantages. Each option brings a gain and a loss. Learn as much as you can about all options. Finally, only you know which is best for you.

You are also in control over the choices you make with regards to your relationships, education, going for help, and keeping yourself healthy physically and mentally. The decisions you make will have a big impact on your future, so consider how these will affect your life and your goals.

Young women have told me that when they found out they were pregnant, it felt as if their life had come to an end. They did not know where to turn for help, and they were faced with all sorts of fears. Judy said: " I was in the darkest tunnel, and saw no light at the end of it."

Have you ever gone through a phase where you just let yourself go? Perhaps you have been looking after yourself, eating healthily and exercising regularly, and then you suddenly find yourself out of control, not working out, eating junk food and gaining too much weight? You remain in this stage for quite a while, because you've sunk too low and it seems like too much effort to turn the situation around.

Then one day you say to yourself, I'm going to do something about this, and you decide that that day you will go to the gym. You've taken one small step. You suddenly feel as if you are a different person. You have taken control of your life and your situation again.

I understand that teenage pregnancy is much more serious than losing control over your dietary and exercise habits, but I want to make a point that taking even that first little step towards regaining control over your life in any situation can make you feel so much stronger.

Sheila, about whom I wrote earlier, took control of her life. Unfortunately she did not get the support she needed from her partner, but she knew she did not have much influence over his decision. Instead, she did have control over her actions, and that was where she was going to put her energy. She had her unborn baby to think of, and she had a career and a future to consider. What she did not have was a lot of money, so she sat down, reviewed her situation, and came up with a financial plan. This plan involved her transferring to another school and moving in with her parents to cut costs. She took many extra little jobs to pay the bills—she tutored, and helped out in a neighborhood bookstore whenever she could.

Remember Maria, who was unable to make a decision, speak to anyone or go for the help she needed because of fear and depression? Well, she too decided to take control of her life. She found that there is always someone to talk to and something one can do to help the situation. She also found that she could still be in control of her life.

Once she spoke to her mother, she was relieved that she was not going to be "thrown out of the house." She found her mother to be more supportive than she had expected. She scheduled the appointment with the obstetrician, and this time was able to listen to her options more calmly. She was given a number of resources, and lots of material to read, and told to take some time to make this important decision. Maria took some time, but knew all along what she wanted to do. After a long family discussion, it was decided that she would raise her baby, with the help of her parents and her aunt, who lived close to their home. Today, Maria is 19 years old, and is a single mother who is making ends meet. She graduated from high school, has a part-time job, and hopes to further her career later. Looking back, she is completely satisfied with the choice she made.

What can you do, here and now, to take control? First, tell yourself that you can't change the past, but from today on you will take control of your future.

The next thing you should do is ask for help. You are not a failure if you ask for help when you need it. You will still be the one to make the final decisions about your pregnancy options.

Where to Turn for Help

STEP ONE: TAKE A PREGNANCY TEST

If you suspect that you are pregnant, confirm this, either by having a blood or urine pregnancy test (beta HCG) done. Symptoms of pregnancy may be vague and nonspecific, so it is important not to rely on symptoms alone. The most obvious symptom of pregnancy is missing a period, but some women develop bleeding as the embryo implants itself in the uterus, and this may be confused with a period. Other common symptoms of early pregnancy are: tiredness, nausea or vomiting, breast tenderness, or frequent urination.

You can have a beta HCG done at a health care facility, or by buying a home pregnancy kit and performing a urine pregnancy test at home, and then confirming the results with your doctor.

STEP TWO: CONFIDE IN SOMEONE

Ideally you would communicate with your parents, the birth father, and possibly other family members. Parents are usually supportive and their involvement can be very helpful. If this is not an option, you may speak to an adult family member, counselor, teacher, or member of the clergy, who can point you in the right direction and offer you support. However, be careful—consider who can be trusted if you want to keep this secret. Your friends may not be mature enough to keep confidences. Most pregnant teenagers are terrified to tell their parents. As one 16-year-old girl told me: "If I tell my Mom she'll kill me!" She finally agreed to let me mediate a meeting between herself and her dad, which I did, and then together we discussed the situation with her mother, and eventually received the support of both.

STEP THREE: SEE A DOCTOR

Do schedule an appointment with a physician as soon as possible. You may begin by seeing your primary care doctor—your internist or pediatrician, who will refer you to an obstetrician as necessary. Teenagers may be more comfortable talking to their pediatricians, especially if they have developed a long-term doctor-patient relationship over the years.

Here are some things a doctor can do for you:

• confirm the results and examine you to make sure that you are healthy. It is important to diagnose the pregnancy as soon as possible, not only so that you can consider the various options, but also so that you can obtain early medical care.

• give you information about options available to you. None of the options is necessarily ideal. Even if you think you have come to a decision, obtain complete information on all available options in order to make a well-informed choice.

• if necessary, mediate between you and your significant others to give them important medical information as well as provide support for all.

• give you information about maintaining your health; i.e., exercise and a healthy diet, and abstaining from tobacco, alcohol, illicit drugs and certain medications.

Alcohol consumed during pregnancy can lead to complications including having a baby with "fetal alcohol syndrome," associated with facial anomalies, retarded growth and nervous system abnormalities. No one is certain about the quantity of alcohol that may be harmful, so it is best to avoid alcohol completely. Smoking tobacco during pregnancy can lead to problems, including having a smaller than normal baby.

• talk about monitoring your health and follow-up visits. Regular prenatal care can greatly reduce your risk of pregnancy-related complications.

• answer any other questions you might have.

• give you a list of resources and support groups in your area. (In Chapter 12 of this book, I do list a number of resources.)

Taking Control No Matter What Your Situation

Your options if you are pregnant include:

• Parenting—with or without a partner.
• Adoption.
• Abortion.

Questions to ask yourself before you make your decision include:

• Which choice could I live with?
• Is there a choice I absolutely could not live with?

- Do I have all the information I need to make my decision?
- How would each choice affect my day-to-day life?
- How would each choice affect the people close to me?

Talk about your feelings to a counselor, a family member, or another trusted adult. Look for a health care provider or a clinic that will give you complete information on all your options. Some clinics do not offer abortion services or counseling, for example. You can also call your local Planned Parenthood Affiliate.

Remember, *you must decide quickly.* If there is a chance that you will continue your pregnancy, you should see a doctor or other qualified health care provider and begin prenatal care as soon as possible. If you are considering abortion, you should decide early, as the risks of abortion increase the longer you wait, and after a certain time in the pregnancy an abortion can no longer be done.

You may be in a situation that makes a decision more difficult. Even so, you can still take control. It helps to be aware of your options. Here are a few situations that may occur, and some suggestions for dealing with them.

ABUSE

Unfortunately, there are many instances in which young people are forced to have sex against their will. Pregnancies can sometimes result from sexual abuse. Some pregnant teenagers are physically or emotionally abused; if you are a victim of rape, incest, or any abuse, it is important to get help immediately. Go to someone you can trust—your doctor, a counselor, a teacher, or another trusted adult. You can also call the Rape, Abuse and Incest National Network Hotline at 1-800-656-HOPE.

RUNAWAYS

If you have run away from home, and cannot return because of abuse or violence or fear, there is help. Some programs include a home for expectant mothers and a facility to care for mothers and their children. You can go to a local clinic, a shelter for runaway teenagers, or a home for pregnant teenagers. As bad as the situation seems now, don't make it worse by not getting help. Your local health care department should be able to help you find out about a shelter.

Kathleen, an 18-year-old patient of mine, came in one day complaining of side effects, including nausea, from an antibiotic prescribed to her at a clinic. On further discussion of her history and after an examination, we found that the nausea was due to pregnancy. Kathleen was in a very difficult and unusual situation. She was in an emotionally and physically abusive relationship with a 22-year-old man, who had coerced her into leaving her home and living with him and his mother. Both her boyfriend and his mother were very controlling, and Kathleen started becoming more withdrawn and losing a lot of weight.

Her mother made calls to the police, and even though they did make a visit to the house, they reported that there was nothing they could do because she was staying there of her own free will. Kathleen made no contact with her mother although they had had a good relationship in the past. She did, however, keep her appointments with me, and slowly she opened up. She was being emotionally controlled by this man, and felt terrified to leave. As luck would have it, he was called to military duty, and when he left, we were able to get her back to her mother's house, and taken care of.

Many women stay in abusive situations for all sorts of reasons that are difficult to understand. Often the male partner is apologetic, and the woman is hopeful he'll change. In other cases, he may threaten her. Don't delay in getting the help you need.

Drug Use

If you are using illegal drugs during your pregnancy, you are causing harm to yourself and your baby. I have mentioned the dangers of alcohol during pregnancy. Smoking can cause problems, including having a baby that is smaller than normal. Other drugs can cause addiction in both the mother and the newborn baby. Injection of drugs can cause HIV infection. Some prescription drugs, such as tetracycline and accutane used for acne, can have side effects during pregnancy, so check with your doctor if you are taking any medications.

What NOT to Do

Don't Despair

Even though this is a very difficult situation, it is not the end of the world, and it is not the end of your life. Millions of teenagers have been faced with unwanted pregnancies and have survived, and even at times gone on to accomplish great things.

DON'T DO THIS ALONE

You may not want to face many people right now, but you cannot deal with everything by yourself, and you will feel much better if you have the support of people you love. Speak to someone you trust and get the help you need.

DON'T PUNISH YOURSELF FURTHER

- Don't neglect your health and well-being.
- Don't withdraw from your family and friends.
- Don't try to hurt yourself.
- Don't use illegal drugs.

DON'T RUN AWAY

At a time like this, it may seem easier to run away, but your problems will stay with you and you will only compound them. If you are in an abusive situation, however, get the help you need to leave, or find out about a shelter in your area.

DON'T RELY ON PEOPLE WHO ARE NOT HELPING YOU

If you don't feel comfortable with the advice you are getting from someone, seek other advice and help.

DON'T LET ANYONE ABUSE YOU

Don't stay with someone who is abusing you, either physically or emotionally. If someone is abusing you, it is *never* your fault. Get help right away.

4

Parenting

"No ordinary work done by a man is either as hard or as responsible as the work of a woman who is bringing up a family of small children; for upon her time and strength demands are made not only every hour of the day but often every hour of the night."
—Theodore Roosevelt (1858–1919)

Even though sexually active teenagers today, compared with those 20 years ago, are more likely to use contraception and less likely to get pregnant, almost one million teenagers do become pregnant in the United States every year and about half carry their babies to term.

Pregnant teenagers today are more likely to give birth to their babies and less likely to give their babies up for adoption, than those 20 years ago. This is partly due to the fact that today there is less social stigma attached to single motherhood. In the 1950s to early 1970s, it was less acceptable to be a single mother. Also, in past generations teenage mothers used to try to do "the right thing" by marrying the baby's father, but today, with younger teenage mothers, this is less realistic. About three-quarters of teenage moms who give birth are unmarried at the time.

Pregnancy and childbirth are major events in any woman's life, but they can be particularly overwhelming when they occur at a young age. As a teenage parent you may have to deal with a wide variety of stresses; e.g., single parenthood, divorce and financial pressures, amongst others. You will also experience many physical and emotional changes. Changes will most likely occur in your relationships with family members and friends. You will need to seriously think about and make decisions about financial matters, your education, your family and your future. There are a number of resources available to you. If you do not know where to look for help, a good start would be your primary physician.

What Are the Primary Responsibilities of Parents?

Parents need to nurture their children and protect them from harm. They need to provide a stimulating environment for them to grow and learn in. They also need to prepare them to become well-adjusted, independent human beings and good members of the community. The quality of parenting, especially of young children, has a great influence on a child's development, both educational and social. For example, children do better with parents who show warmth and sensitivity towards them and provide reasonable guidance and structure, rather than being too harsh and rigid. You may or may not have had a good role model for parenting. In either case you need to be a good role model to your child. I don't think it's true that some people are not destined to be good parents. Parenting skills can be taught. One third of all children born in the U.S. are born to never married parents, so there is much interest in teaching skills to those parents. Parent education can help you become a better parent. Your doctor or local health department can help you find classes available to you.

Carrie was 15 when she gave birth to Peter. I met her when she was 16 and pregnant for the second time. Carrie was still dating her boyfriend of two years and she believed that marriage was in their future. She would have liked to delay motherhood, but when she became pregnant, she knew that she wanted to take care of her baby. Neither abortion nor adoption was an option for her. Carrie does parent her little boy with a lot of help from her mother, with whom they live. "It's tough being a single mom, but we're managing. I love my son Peter and I definitely want to be a mother to my second baby too."

I recently visited a transitional housing program for single young mothers. The program provides a supportive environment for young mothers while they finish school or go to work. Many teenage mothers can't find a job because they have no training. They can't get training or finish school because they have a baby to care for and no money for day care or a sitter. One of the missions of the program is to prepare young mothers to become self-supporting effective parents.

I met with about ten young mothers living there with their children, who ranged in age from one to two years. This arrangement allows them to work at an outside job during the day, knowing that their children will be cared for. When they return from work, they are expected to resume all normal responsibilities, including cooking for themselves and their children and studying if required. Life is not easy for them, they reminded me, but they have food and clothing and an opportunity to build a better future. They support each other during their difficult times and celebrate their accomplishments together. One of the happiest moments was when one of the graduates of the program married after leaving, and returned to the residence to celebrate her wedding.

Lina was 18 when she became pregnant. She was in a steady relationship with a man she was sure she would marry. She used no contraception and in fact wasn't too upset about her pregnancy, as a baby fitted nicely into her plans for the future. Soon after she delivered her baby, however, her boyfriend left her, and her world crumbled. Through a family friend, she heard about this transitional housing program, where she now lives with her one-year-old son. Lina has learned from her past. She is in no hurry to date again and she knows that one of the biggest mistakes she could make now would be to become pregnant for the second time. Her dream is to become a psychologist, although at this stage it is still very hard for Lina to see past bottle feedings, diaper changes and sleepless nights.

The second young mother I met was Ruth, who became pregnant at the age of 19. She believed that everything would fall into place when she married her boyfriend. Unfortunately it didn't turn out that way at all. Jake left her even before she delivered, and has nothing to do with his baby girl, leaving Ruth to care for her alone. Ruth never considered adoption—"no-one spoke about it"—and does not believe in abortion, so deciding to parent was a natural choice for her. "Here we're all struggling, but it's like a family. We pay rent and day-care fees and learn to budget. The program has made me more responsible and given me a safe place to stay with my baby while I work to support the two of us."

Pros and Cons of Parenting

First, let us look at the good things about parenting.

• By not giving them to someone else to raise, you will be able to raise your own child.

• You will feel a sense of pride as you develop and prove your parenting skills.

• You can share in shaping you child's future and watch as they grow and reach new milestones.

• You will love someone who will love you in return.

• Children give you more rewards than you can ever imagine.

There are, however, a lot of difficulties. Here are a few:

• You need a lot of stamina. Babies require attention 24 hours a day.
• You'll be faced with adult problems—for example, financial problems—at an early age.
• Your life will change. You will have less freedom, and less time to spend with friends and to go to movies and so on.
• It will be more difficult to finish school.
• It will be more difficult to continue with your career. You may have to put things on hold for a while.

If you decide to parent your child, ask yourself the following:

• What are my reasons for wanting to be a parent now?
• Do I understand the responsibility required to be a parent? Babies need attention up to 24 hours a day. They can never be left alone.
• Can I handle the stress of taking care of a colicky baby night after night? This is a full time commitment.
• Am I emotionally and financially ready to parent a child?
• Where will I live?
• Do I have health insurance for myself and the baby?
• Will I be able to buy food, clothes and diapers?

With changes in the welfare laws, government support will no longer be automatic.

Do you have a strong support system in place? Ideally you would have the support of your family and the baby's father. Studies show, for example, that children develop better when a supportive grandparent is involved, than if a teenage mother is isolated while raising her child. It is a good idea, therefore, to involve your parents in the lives of your children, if they are caring and supportive.

It may also be a good idea to join a teenage parent support group in your area. Many types of support groups exist. They offer education and opportunities for networking and sharing experiences with others. Check with your physician or counselor for a recommendation.

How Will Having a Baby Change My Life?

Lifestyle and Relationship Changes

As a young mother, you may at times experience intense highs—joy and excitement—and at other times extreme lows, with periods of stress and anxiety. Pregnant teenagers who choose parenting over abortion or adoption, sometimes do so to avoid the feeling of "loss"; however, even parenting is associated with some loss. Changes in relationships are likely to occur with your family, your baby's father and even your friends. It may be hard to relate to your friends who aren't pregnant or don't have children. Some won't approve of the decisions you have made. You may want to spend time with family or friends, but find there is too much to juggle. Raising your baby requires you to be responsible for that child 24 hours a day. Babies need constant attention, feedings and diaper changes, and you may find that you don't have energy for much else at first. This can result in a sense of loss, not spending time with friends, missing out on social functions and even school and career opportunities. No, you will not have to give up on all your activities and friends. It just means that you will have to be organized and prioritize. Of course your baby comes first.

Carol had to live with a friend while she raised her baby. "It's harder than I ever thought it would be," she said. "I have no freedom." Many young mothers live at home with their parents. If this is the case with you, think about what role you'd like your parents to play in the raising of your child. Remember that moving in with your parents requires an adjustment for them as well as for you, so be appreciative. If you do need to borrow money from your parents, do it in a businesslike manner, and make sure you attempt to pay back what you owe them.

On the other hand parenting and raising a baby can be very rewarding. Seeing your baby grow and reach milestones, such as giving a first smile or taking a first step, can be very exciting. Raising a child has given some teenagers an incentive to do better in life. As Debbie said: "My life has meaning now. I feel as if I've accomplished something."

CHANGES IN YOUR EDUCATION

As a teenage mother your chances of graduating from high school these days are much higher than they were in the 1970s. Many schools are making it easier for teenage mothers to attend classes, and some schools even have on-site daycare. The good news is that a teenage mother who has her baby while she's in school, who is able to stay in school, and has a good support system, has a good chance of graduating. On the other hand, teenage mothers often find it difficult to stay in school, are less likely to attend college, are less likely to obtain high-paying jobs, and, therefore, are more likely to be poor. The responsibilities of being a teenage mother can be overwhelming, especially if you are single. So many teenage mothers rely on their families or on public assistance payments for financial support.

How can you continue your education after you give birth?:

• You may be lucky enough to be able to live at home with your parents, and have them take care of your baby while you are in school. If you have this arrangement it is important for you to do your share. Offer to do a job to earn money so that you can pay some rent. Help with housework or other chores. And remember, this is a big adjustment for them too.

• You may need a daycare situation—a sitter to come to your home, a family child-care service, or a daycare center—so that you can attend classes.

• Some schools or colleges might offer on-site daycare.

• You might consider at-home schooling or evening classes.

• You may make an arrangement for a friend or family member to look after your child a few days a week while you attend part-time classes.

CHANGES IN YOUR FINANCES

Money isn't everything, but life certainly becomes a little easier when you have enough money to pay the monthly bills and have some left over for emergencies and a few "extras." Being a single mother makes it more difficult to earn a decent income, and raising a baby is expensive. You will need to buy food, clothes, diapers, and toys, and there are also medical bills and health insurance to consider. Of course, it doesn't stop there, because as your baby gets older, you'll need money for schooling, transportation, babysitters and much more. Many teenage mothers remain single and get no support from the father of their child. They must support themselves and their babies, often with the help of their families. Although many teenage moms have to struggle financially, they do, with hard work and perseverance, overcome these hardships. However, you cannot do this on your own. You will need a strong support system. This support may come from your baby's father, your family, another responsible adult or a teenage mother "support group."

Here are some tips for managing your finances:

• The first step to managing your finances is to be honest about and to take control over your money situation, no matter how bad things look.

• Make a budget. Prioritize your expenses.

• Don't use credit cards. Don't get yourself into debt. If you are in debt, pay it off as soon as you can.

• Write down your short-term and long-term goals.

• Save wherever you can. Before you can think about saving, though, it's important to know what you spend.

• Keep a record of your expenses for two or three months and see what your fixed and optional expenses are each month. Fixed expenses would include rent, utilities and medical expenses. Optional expenses are things like household items, gifts and entertainment.

Saving money is difficult, but here are some possibilities to consider:

• Living with your parents while your baby is young can help with saving money as well as providing you with emotional support. Remember that even though this may not be your first choice, it will probably be an adjustment for your parents too. Your parents may have become used to the freedom and quiet of living on their own and if you move in with your child, although they may be happy, this could create quite a lifestyle change for them.

• It's important to establish paternity. Make sure your baby's father is helping with costs through child-support payments.

• Consider sharing babysitting with other young mothers.

• Earn extra money by working at home. Women today are starting many successful new businesses.

• You may qualify for public assistance. Check with your social services or local health care department.

• The Department of Social Services may help with money, food stamps, medical assistance and child-support enforcement if you qualify. You will probably be eligible for WIC (Women, Infants and Children), a federal program which provides healthy foods to pregnant, breastfeeding and postpartum women, and to infants and children under age five. Your local health department can provide information on services available and may offer free immunizations, counseling and other care.

• Check on scholarships for college.

• Even though it costs some money, having insurance, including life, disability, health and car insurance, will probably save you a lot of money in the long run.

You may be worried about losing your job if you're pregnant. You should know that the Pregnancy Discrimination Act (1978) says that pregnant women must be treated in the same way as other applicants or employees of similar ability. In addition, if you need to be absent from work because of a pregnancy-related condition, your employer must hold open your job for the same length of time as the job would be held open for employees on sick or disability leave.

Should I Be a Parent with or Without a Partner?

You have more options to consider once you have decided to raise your baby. You can marry, or stay single and raise your baby on your own with or without the support of the baby's father. In the early 1960s, only about a third of first time teenage mothers remained single, but today more than three-quarters choose to do so. The average teenage mother today is younger, and single motherhood is more accepted than it was in the past.

Two-Parent Families

Marriage has advantages and disadvantages. The downside is that teenage marriage is often a temporary solution. More than half of teenage marriages fail, and marriage does not guarantee that your spouse will be emotionally supportive. There is a good side to marriage too. Most women would eventually like to find a partner with whom to share the rest of their lives. If you have a good relationship with the baby's father, he will be a support for you and the baby, and you will have someone who can share the responsibilities and help financially, and your baby will have the advantage of growing up with both parents.

Remember, though, that marriage is a serious legal contract, and you must decide if marriage is right for you both at this time. If marriage is your choice, consider premarital counseling. If both of you are committed to making it work, and you know each other's expectations, the marriage has a much greater chance of succeeding.

Single Parent Families

You may decide that marriage is not right for you at this time, or circumstances may have dictated that for you. What was once considered the norm in America—a two-parent family, with an employed father and a stay-at-home mother—is no longer so in the new millennium. About half of all children spend several years in a single-parent household because of divorce, death of a spouse, or parents not marrying.

For a number of reasons, some young men leave a relationship after they learn that their partner is pregnant. They often do so because they can't or don't want to deal with the responsibility of a child. Your partner may say he is not ready to parent, he may try to coerce you into having an abortion, or he may be ambivalent about his feelings and leave the decisions up to you. Many young men are truly afraid and may not know fully what is expected of them.

Do establish paternity, unless you are positive that you don't want the father to be a part of your lives, either emotionally or financially. Hopefully he will take responsibility and acknowledge that he is the baby's father. If your baby's father is not abusive and wants to be involved, it's best not to deny him access to his child, even though he has decided not to stay with you.

If he has decided to leave, accept this. Don't torture yourself with the notion that you are inadequate or that you caused him to leave. This is probably not the case. There are usually more complex reasons involved when fathers walk away, so there is no need to blame yourself. Be honest with yourself about how you feel about your situation and the loss of the relationship. Do get help if you feel persistent or overwhelming sadness or you need someone to talk this over with. Now is the time for you to take responsibility for yourself and your baby.

Even though statistics reveal that a single-parent family is at higher risk for lower family income, behavioral problems, and social isolation, these problems are not inevitable. Single motherhood, as a result of women being divorced, widowed, or unmarried, is becoming more common, so it's important to take a look at ways in which mothers in this situation can do the best for their children.

We have learned that in general, children do best with both a mother and father present. As we have seen, this is not always possible and many young women have done a remarkable job of raising their children on their own, with help from family members and friends. Many children who have grown up in single-parent families have thrived and become successful, and this is largely due to the fact that children can form close attachments to grandparents, aunts or uncles, or other loving adults, when their parents are absent.

For a single mother, raising children can be very tough. Getting the children to school, picking them up, preparing meals, putting them to bed, buying clothes, and paying bills, can cause great emotional stress at times. Children can make her miss work and keep her from social activities. They can develop physical and emotional problems. They can also prevent her from dating.

On the other hand, children bring meaning to her life. They are energetic and challenging. They can provide healthy distractions when she needs it most, and they are there to love her and receive love from her in return.

We must not forget that fathers have feelings too. For the father, who may only see his child occasionally, the emotional and financial pressures are stressful, and often he may feel a deep sense of loss about not being part of an intact family.

However, if the parents can successfully juggle the schedules involved with taking care of themselves and the children, the family has an excellent chance of surviving and sometimes thriving. A working mother who is successfully taking care of the bills, feeding her children and educating them, often feels a sense of accomplishment.

It is important to take care of your own needs too, so that you can better help the family. Don't be afraid to ask for help. When problems are overwhelming, it is not a sign of weakness to ask a relative or a friend to help you. You can also seek professional help from your doctor or a counselor. Keeping to routines can be helpful.

How else can a single mother do the best for her child or children? In the case of divorce and a father who cares about his children, or a young unmarried father who would like to be involved, the mother can encourage visitation and contact between father and children as often as possible. This way the children can still have some of the benefits of having both parents, even if they are not living together. Being a single mother can be overwhelming at times. You don't have a father who can regularly help with feeding, transport, putting the children to bed, or disciplining them. But it is not necessary to be a martyr; it is okay to ask for help. Your children will do better if more loving caretakers are involved. So, if necessary, move in with your parents for a while until you feel more stable. Having the love and involvement of their grandparents can go a long way in helping children of single parents gain self-esteem and feel loved.

You will need to consider financial issues, child-care arrangements, and whether you will be going to school or working, among other things. Dating or going out with friends can become complicated. You will learn a lot about parenting and managing your time as you go along, but it's a good idea to ask for help if needed and to speak to your doctor or health care provider about parenting issues. As a new mother you may also ask about parenting classes. In these classes you will most likely learn about topics such as feeding your baby, teaching, and safety issues. Many questions can also be answered in the hospital after delivery; questions, for instance, on breast versus bottle feeding, bathing and diaper changing, and how to choose a doctor for your baby.

What to tell your child: As a single parent you may wonder how and when to talk to you child about your situation. Every situation is unique, and what's right for one person may not be right for another. What is important, though, is honesty. It is okay to explain to your child that you have made mistakes in the past, but have learned from them. Always reassure your child how much you love them.

Emotions: You will probably have some strong emotional ups and downs. One emotion you'll probably encounter is grief. Every single mother goes through some form of grieving process, because she has lost something. She has lost the chance to have an intact family and a life partner, her innocence, and perhaps an opportunity to further her education and career at this time. You need to know that it is normal to have some of these feelings, as long as you can work through them. If you are unable to resolve them and do not reach a stage of acceptance, you must get help.

Another emotion is guilt. Many single mothers feel a lot of guilt. They feel guilty about being a single parent without a full-time father for their children. They feel guilty about not having enough money to provide all the material things they would like to provide for their children. Some mothers overcompensate because of guilt, and may become overly permissive parents. This creates more problems. The important thing to remember is that children value your time and attention much more than "things" in the long run. Ask almost any child if they would rather have a toy, or have Mommy come home from work to spend time with them. The best you can do is show your children love, and help them feel good about themselves.

Self-esteem. Your child's self-esteem will play an important role in how they develop as a person, perform in school and work, and interact with other people. People with low self-esteem feel unimportant and unworthy. Even if you are a single parent, you can still help your children develop high self-esteem.

- Always treat your children with dignity and respect.
- Make them feel important and worthy, and let them know that their feelings count.

- Respect their opinions.
- Encourage them to help others (this will give them a sense of accomplishment).
- Spend time with them (quality and quantity counts).
- Praise them for accomplishments—big and little.
- Make them feel secure.

Discipline: Children need someone to be in control and make certain decisions for them. They need to feel that there are some limits and that someone cares enough to set those limits. You need to be that person. Disciplining children is more difficult for single moms because they don't have a partner to reinforce their authority, and they have no one to hand things over to when they become frustrated and tired.

Discipline is not synonymous with punishment. The goal of discipline should be teaching and learning consequences. You can use the following methods, among others, instead of screaming, spanking or losing control.

• Time out: Separating yourself from your child gives your child time to think about what they did, and you time to cool off.

• Taking away privileges: If the bad behavior continues, taking away a privilege such as television can be effective.

• Teaching consequences: Having to do a certain chore if a rule is broken, for example, can be used.

If you are still struggling with discipline and nothing seems to work, ask your pediatrician, a therapist, or school counselor for help.

Developing independence: The children of single mothers are often more independent than children who live with their mom and dad together. They have to be. They need to help their mother with tasks such as preparing lunch for school, chores around the home, or washing the car, because there is only so much she can do alone. Single parents must be careful not to expect too much from their children. They are not adults and should not have to take on the role and responsibility of another parent.

Dating again: At a certain point in time, you will probably want to start dating again, although one young woman I spoke to said she never wanted to talk to a man again. How she felt was understandable. Her boyfriend, Jake, left her when he learned that she was pregnant, came back into her life three months later, and is now in prison. She will not say why.

Not all men are like Jake by any means, but it is still wise to wait a while until you start dating again. Your children need your time and attention now more than ever, and you need to decide what you want out of life and to make plans for the future for yourself and your children. As you start dating, I don't think it's wise to introduce your children to every man you date. Your children have suffered the loss of a full-time father already, and they don't need more unnecessary losses.

Lynn had her first child at the age of 17. She has had no contact with the father since. She married at the age of 19 and had a second baby. When her second child, Jason, was a year old, she divorced, and was left with two young children with no father. When she met Derek, she felt as if her prayers had been answered. He seemed to love her children. He helped with driving, cooking, and putting them to bed. He earned a good salary, and it was not long before he moved in with Lynn and the children. Marriage wasn't really discussed, but Lynn believed it was inevitable. She couldn't complain for now. The children were becoming very attached to Derek. Eighteen months later, the relationship ended. Now it was a terrible loss not only for the couple, but also for the two young children, whose security had been taken away from them.

Counseling for single parents: There are a large number of groups across the U.S. that help single parents and provide counseling. Experienced counselors will listen to you and help you deal with the problems of being a single parent. As a single parent, you may not know what is expected of you or where to turn for help, so it can be of considerable benefit to receive guidance about how to provide for yourself and your child. Counselors can help answer questions such as the following:

- What are my rights and responsibilities as a single parent?
- What is child support?
- How do I establish paternity?
- How can I get to see my child more often?

Counseling can be one on one, or with family members, or in groups. Support groups are also a form of counseling. You will be part of a group of people who have been in similar situations.

THE WORKING MOTHER

You may want to stay at home with your children while they are very young, so that you can care for them and watch them develop. Lack of finances can make this very difficult, but you can always find a way to manage.

• Living with your parents may not be a good long-term plan, but it can be a satisfactory short-term solution. It can be an opportunity for you as a single mother to save some money to buy or rent an apartment or to pay off bills.
• Some single mothers live off welfare checks in spite of the financial and psychological burden.
• Often women find they are able to earn a living by working at home.
• You may take a part-time job outside of the home, to earn some income, but also spend time with your kids.

In an ideal situation, you would have enough money to be able to stay at home with your children while they are young, and perhaps work part-time from home; or your parents could baby-sit while you worked, so that you would not have to hire a babysitter or put your children in daycare.

However, this is not always the case, and many single mothers find that they don't have any alternatives, other than using some form of child-care.

In-home care is one possibility. There are many advantages to this situation.

• Your baby will be in their own home, and will have more attention in a one-on-one environment with the sitter, rather than being in a group-care setting.
• Children in daycare settings are frequently exposed to respiratory and gastric infections. Because your baby is less exposed to other children in your own home, they will also be less likely to pick up these infections at an early age.
• The other advantage, I think, is that you have more control over what happens in your home. You can set the standards, and you can make unscheduled visits at any time to check on your baby.
• You will not have to commute for child care.

There are also disadvantages to in-home care:

• It may be more expensive.
• Your child may not have interaction with other children. This is usually not a problem in the case of a baby or young child.
• You will have the presence of someone else in your home when you are not there.

If you decide on in-home care, you will have to choose a sitter. This is one of the very important decisions you will make, choosing the person who will be responsible for your baby when you are not there. The sitter may be referred by word of mouth. If someone you trust makes a strong recommendation, this can go a long way to making you feel more secure. You may also find a sitter through an agency, or through an ad in a newspaper or a parenting or school magazine.

Before hiring a sitter:

- Obtain references, on the phone and in writing.
- Do a personal interview.
- Spend at least a day with the sitter, watching the sitter's interaction with your child.
- Make sure that the sitter has basic safety knowledge and is trained in CPR.
- Go over several possible scenarios, and ask how they would react in those situations.

Always have your contact information at home in case you need to be reached. It's also best to have other emergency numbers posted where they are easily visible.

Family daycare is another option. Some women choose to earn extra money looking after children in their own homes, while caring for their own children at the same time. There are good and bad points with this type of arrangement. This is sometimes cheaper than a daycare center or a private sitter, and usually there are fewer children in a private home than in a center, so theoretically your child could receive more attention. On the other hand, the caregiver may not be very experienced in looking after children. Last year a friend of mine had placed her baby in a family care setting. She had to take her baby out after one week, as the caregiver was overwhelmed by her own child's needs, and really couldn't cope with looking after another baby too.

Daycare centers are a very common form of child care. Here are some tips for choosing a daycare center:

- Make sure the center is licensed and in good standing.
- Get references and recommendations from friends and acquaintances.
- Visit the center. Check on cleanliness.
- Interview the director of the facility to discuss their philosophies.
- Ask about their policies on discipline, and infection control.
- Ask about the training of the caregivers.

• Make sure that you are allowed to make unannounced visits at any time.

At-work daycare is sometimes available. Some companies provide on-site childcare, though this is still rare.

A young single mother I know works as an executive assistant for a large company. She is an outstanding worker and an outstanding mother. They obviously recognized her talents and her devotion to her work and her daughter. They therefore made a special allowance for her, and she brings her daughter to work every day, in spite of there being no formal office daycare policy. Clearly, this could not be a solution for all types of jobs, but for Kerry it is a dream come true. She makes a good living and is able to see her beautiful daughter whenever she wishes.

With so many single parents in the work force, I really wish that more businesses and corporations would consider on-site daycare. They need to know that happy parents, parents who are not worrying about their children, will make much better employees and will be more productive. A few large companies have recognized this need, and have started a trend, but we still have a long way to go.

Working at home is sometimes possible. If you are lucky enough to be able to work at home, here are some of the advantages:

• You are able to spend more time with your children and can be available in case of emergencies.
• The hours are flexible.
• You will save money on childcare.
• You do not have to commute to work.
• There are fewer "office" interruptions.

There are also disadvantages to working at home:

• You will need to be very motivated.
• It may be distracting working around your children.
• Office support services and staff are not available.

Here are some possible options for work at home (this is only a small list; other options may be available):

• Childcare.
• Typing, editing, computer programming.

- Writing.
- Tutoring.
- Teaching languages, music, and so on.
- Operating a small business from home.
- Accounting.
- Telemarketing.

Child Abuse and Neglect

I recently saw a young baby, the son of a 17-year-old unmarried mother. He had been abused by his biological father, and had suffered a severe head injury from "shaken baby syndrome." Shaken baby syndrome is the result of a whiplash-type injury from shaking a baby violently. This can result in serious brain damage and visual problems.

Until all the circumstances are sorted out, he will stay with a foster parent and then hopefully be returned to his mother and grandmother. His father is currently in prison. What a sad situation, and one that is preventable. If you suspect abuse or feel excessively stressed, ask for help right away.

Most abusing parents are not psychotic and don't have criminal personalities (*Nelson Textbook of Pediatrics*). They are usually lonely, unhappy, angry and very stressed. They have often themselves experienced physical abuse as children.

If you start to get serious about a man, be sure that he relates well to your children and that you can trust him. When a single mother lives with a man, this man may or may not have the best interests of her children at heart. The first function of a mother must be to protect her children from harm, and this includes abuse from anyone. If you suspect that emotional, physical, or sexual abuse is occurring, even if the children seem to be coping with it, you've got to report this and get help right away.

Not all single-parent homes are doomed by any means. In many cases single-parent families have very positive outcomes. Single parenting allows the development of the parent's independence and ability to handle difficult situations, and also allows them to practice making good decisions. In addition, it allows children to develop increased levels of responsibility. Good communication between parent and child and between the two parents, improves the outcome even further.

Choosing a Pediatrician for Your Baby

Babies require a lot of health care in the first two years, when you take into account their routine physicals and immunization visits, as well as any sick visits that may be needed. For this reason, it is wise to choose a pediatrician whom you trust and with whom you can communicate easily.

Many pediatricians offer a free prenatal appointment, which means that you can meet with a prospective pediatrician and decide if they will be a good match for you.

What are some of the questions you should ask and issues you should consider?

• Are the pediatricians in the group board-certified in pediatrics? This implies that they have had extra training in the field.
• What are the hours of operation of the practice? Are they open on Saturdays, early mornings, or evenings?
• What happens if you need an emergency sick appointment? Will you be able to walk in or get an appointment on that day?
• To which hospitals do the pediatricians admit patients, and at which hospitals do they visit and examine newborn patients?
• Is someone from the group available if you have an emergency in the middle of the night or on weekends?
• Does the group participate in your insurance plan?
• Do you agree with the philosophies of the pediatrician?
• Is an advice nurse available in the daytime to call if you have questions?

Caring for Your Newborn

If you make the decision, while you are pregnant, that you will parent your child, you should do some reading on the subject. You may read about what to expect in the hospital and the first few days after you give birth, and what to expect from and how to care for your baby in the first few months. No baby follows the books exactly, but it is useful to know what's normal, so that you can be a little more prepared. Also, check with your pediatrician about available resources and support groups.

Enjoying Your Baby

Don't forget to take time occasionally and just have fun with your baby. The time that I always remember is when my baby was six weeks old. I was sitting in the rocking chair very late at night feeding him, and he suddenly turned and looked right in my face, and smiled. This was his first smile and it was a magical moment. There are many moments like that. It's a pity though that we are so tired when our babies are little that we can't really enjoy many of them or even notice them.

So, take a break sometimes, and watch your baby develop: the first time they roll over, the first laugh, the first word.

Preparing Your Older Child for a Sibling

Assuming you already have a child, and you are pregnant again, there are some things to keep in mind to make the adjustment easier for your older child. I've heard siblings say of their new baby sister or brother: "I don't want her"; or, "He's okay, but can we send him back now?"

An older child who is used to being the center of attention can feel very threatened by a new baby's arrival. He may feel insecure, or even afraid that he is being replaced. Some children seem to regress when the new baby comes along. For example, if they were potty trained, they might start wetting again. If they were weaned off a bottle, they might want the bottle, or a pacifier. Parents need to handle this in a sensitive manner.

• Gradually prepare your older child for the new baby.

• Your child's age and level of curiosity and interest will determine when in your pregnancy you let her know.

• Allow your older child to be involved in some of the preparation.

• Some pediatricians believe that you shouldn't use your older child's crib for the new baby. I think that's probably right, especially if your child has just been weaned from the crib.

• Assure your child that you will not love him or her any less.

• Take advantage of sibling classes offered by some hospitals.

• Your older child should keep to the usual routine as much as possible.

• Spend time with your older child whenever possible. Perhaps occasionally someone else could take over feeding or putting the baby to sleep.

• Let your older child be a "helper," bringing a diaper or the bottle, and give frequent praise.

Staying in Control

Set goals for yourself. Mention that you are a pregnant teenager or a single teenage mother and many people will believe that your destiny has been set and that your future is bleak. However, in spite of statistics, you can control your future. You are the one who makes your choices and you still have the opportunity to make good choices from this point onward.

1. Decide not to become pregnant again, until you are in a committed marriage. A large number of teenage girls have second and even third unwanted pregnancies.

2. When making decisions from now on, always consider the best interests of your child too.

3. Make the decision to be the best parent you can.

4. Get support from your family and friends. Consider living with your parents or other relatives, provided the environment is safe for you and your baby.

5. Enquire about financial aid. A local Planned Parenthood clinic, your doctor, or a school counselor can point you in the right direction.

6. Join a teen parent support group.

7. Decide that you will complete your schooling or further your education, even if you study part-time. A higher education will allow you to find better employment in the future and help with self-esteem.

8. Decide that you will earn money by working part-time, even if you have to work at home for a few hours while your baby sleeps.

It may take time to reach your long-term goals, but picture where you would like to see yourself in the future. Unless you know what your goals are, you won't be able to reach them. Set small goals for yourself in the meantime, so that as you accomplish these you will feel good about yourself. I recommend having a role model, such as a teacher, counselor, friend, or relative you can talk to and who can guide you.

Teenage mothers can be good parents. A good support system can help you accomplish that goal. Don't give up. Continue to set goals for yourself. Being a single parent is one of the toughest challenges in life, but if you put in the time and the effort, you will be rewarded. Thousands of women have not only survived single motherhood, but thrived and accomplished great things in life. With planning and perseverance, you too can raise your children to be happy, healthy and independent people, while still accomplishing your goals and becoming a fulfilled person.

Samantha's Story

I'll never forget Samantha and her parents. I was a pediatric resident working in an intensive care nursery. We cared for a large number of babies in that unit—most of them premature, and some with lung disease or other problems. Samantha was one of my first patients and I came to know her pretty well, as she remained in the unit for about seven months. She was born about 14 weeks early, and her lungs were not well developed, so she needed oxygen and help with her breathing for a long time. She also developed an infection which was treated with antibiotics, and required tube feeding at first as she was unable to suck.

Her parents spent most of every day at her crib, helping with her feeding, learning from the nurses and supporting each other. I often watched them and admired how they handled the situation. In spite of her many problems, with the care she received from the staff and from her parents, Samantha did remarkably well. The nurses became very attached to her, as did I. I laugh when I remember her being our only baby to be eating yogurt in the intensive care unit. She was getting so chubby!

I mentioned before that I took care of so many babies with similar problems, and watched many parents visit their premature infants in the nursery. Why then was this situation different? Samantha's parents were only 15 years old.

Premature babies require constant care and frequent visits to doctors. These young parents made a decision to stay together and parent their baby, in spite of the sacrifices required. They knew they had made a mistake, but decided to take responsibility for the situation and deal with it as best they could. I'll always admire them for that.

Nicole, a young mother of a beautiful two-year-old girl, told me that her boyfriend, Ray, was uninvolved even during her pregnancy. They never discussed their pregnancy options or financial or legal issues. There was no question about whether Nicole would parent. She wanted to be a mother to her child, even though she knew she would be a single mother. I asked Nicole what pregnancy and parenthood changed about her life. "It changes everything one hundred percent! It changes relationships with friends, because you have no time. I was sleep-deprived, so it affected my work. I must say, things have become a lot easier now, though."

Nicole read many books on pregnancy and what to expect during the first years of childhood. She also used resources available to her in her area. This and the fact that her mother was so supportive, saved her, she said. She believes that her daughter has benefited tremendously from having the love of her grandmother and other close friends. Sadly, the father is still rarely present and sees his daughter less than once a month. He has been ordered by the courts to pay child support, but payments are irregular.

I have met Nicole's daughter and seen how happy and well-adjusted she appears to be. I asked Nicole what advice she had for single mothers. She finds it important to surround herself with supportive people. She was helped by having a babysitter that she could really trust, and finds it important to go out occasionally, even two or three times a month, to rejuvenate. "It's also important to know that if you are occasionally stressed out and find yourself thinking that you wish you had never decided to parent, that you are not a bad person. It's normal to have those feelings sometimes."

As I watch Nicole interact with her little daughter, I think that for her, those feelings must be very rare.

Adoption

Raising a child is challenging in many ways, even for a stable couple with a regular income. Until you've spent 48 hours in charge of an infant by yourself, you can't imagine how hard it is to be a parent. Most adolescents don't have the resources available to be able to raise a child on their own. I recently interviewed 30-year-old Kayla, who is now a wonderful mother to her three-year-old daughter. She looks back upon the time when she was 19 and pregnant for the first time, and doesn't know how she would have managed. She believes she made the right decision by choosing adoption at that time.

Study after study shows that it is ideal for a child to be raised in a two-parent loving family. It may be surprising to you then that the number of teenage mothers who place their babies for adoption is so low—far fewer than a generation ago. There is not much information on the exact number, but between 1989 and 1995, just under one percent of babies born to never-married women were placed for adoption (*ChildTrends* 1995). The number has fallen dramatically from over eight percent before 1970. To put this in perspective, each year over 300,000 of the million teenage pregnancies end in induced abortion, while about 6,000 babies are placed for adoption. One of the reasons for the low number of adoptions is that although single motherhood is still hard, it's no longer a "disgrace"—and some women are very successful despite the difficulties. Other reasons for the decreased number of babies available for adoption are the ready availability of contraception and the legalization of abortion in 1973. As a result, there are more couples waiting to adopt babies.

Why Do Women Choose Adoption?

Sometimes, unfortunately, a pregnancy occurs at a time when you know you are unable to support a child and unable to offer what the child needs. One of the most common reasons for placing a child for adoption is not feeling emotionally ready to parent a child at the time. Some feel they cannot provide for a child at the time. If the father is not in the picture, the birthmother may choose adoption so that the baby can have both a mother and father present. Some opt for adoption because they feel that parenting at the time would affect their education or career.

If you know that you are unable to raise your baby and you believe that abortion is not the right choice—for religious, moral or other reasons—adoption is the option for you. The baby will be raised by adults who are screened, qualified, and eager to be parents, if you go through a reputable adoption agency. There is evidence that children adopted in infancy do about as well as nonadopted children. As age at adoption increases, problems appear to increase (Sharma et al, 1996).

Terminology

Before continuing, let me define the following terms used in this chapter:

• *Adoptive parents*—the couple that adopts the baby.
• *Adoptee*—the child who is adopted.
• *Adoption agency*—an organization, usually licensed by the state, that provides services to birthparents, adoptive parents and children who need families. Agencies may be public or private, secular or religious, for profit or nonprofit.
• *Adoption attorney*—a legal professional who has experience with filing, processing, and finalizing adoptions. For an adoption attorney you can contact the American Academy of Adoption Attorneys at 202-832-2222, or you can look in the phone book under "American Bar Association."
• *Adoption facilitator*—an individual whose business involves connecting birthparents and prospective adoptive parents for a fee (not allowed in every state).
• *Adoption placement*—the point at which a child begins to live with prospective adoptive parents; the period before the adoption is finalized.
• *Birthparents*—the biological parents of the child.
• *Closed adoption*—an adoption that involves total confidentiality and sealed records. The birthparents and the adoptive parents never know each other.

• *Consent papers*—the papers that the birthparents sign to waive their rights to parent their child.

• *Independent adoption*—an adoption facilitated by those not associated with an agency. Facilitators may be attorneys, physicians or other intermediaries. Independent adoptions are only legal in certain states.

• *Open adoption*—an adoption that involves some amount of initial or ongoing contact between the birthparents and adoption families.

• ******—a determined amount of time after signing of the consent papers in which the birthparents can reclaim parental rights to their baby. This varies from state to state, and in some states there is no such period.

Advantages and Disadvantages of Adoption

As with anything else, there are advantages and disadvantages to adoption. Here are some of the advantages:

• As a teenager you may not be emotionally ready; nor may you have the resources available to you to raise a child. Adoption allows you to postpone parenting.

• You may disagree with abortion on personal, religious or moral grounds.

• Adoption provides your child the opportunity to have a better life than that which you could provide at this time.

• You will have given the greatest gift and blessing to the adoptive parents, who may not otherwise have had the opportunity of having a child.

• Young birthmothers who postpone parenthood and choose adoption, usually have more education, better job opportunities, and are less likely to have another premarital pregnancy than those who keep their babies.

Disadvantages include the following:

• You still need to experience a complete pregnancy.

• Adoption ends your legal right to parent your child.

• Adoption is associated with feelings of loss, in spite of believing that you are doing what's best for your baby.

• Because adoption is not often considered by young parents, teenagers may find difficulty getting support from their friends.

Making the Adoption Decision

Adoption isn't easy. Before you decide, ask yourself these questions:

- Am I ready to make the decision?
- Have I explored all other possibilities? For example, if I had help financially, would I decide to parent?
- Am I being pressured into the decision by family or friends? It should be your decision.
- Are my parents against the decision?
- Will I work with an adoption agency or an independent source?
- Do I know that I am not ready to parent?
- Am I only considering adoption because of financial problems which may be temporary?

Talking to others can help you resolve these issues. Here are some people who you might be able to talk to:

- Physician.
- Adoption agency.
- Adoption attorney.
- Family planning clinic.
- A crisis pregnancy center.
- Health department or social services.
- A counselor at a mental health center or family service agency.

If you are considering placing your baby for adoption, go through these steps:

1. Speak to family members, the birthfather, or trusted friends, to the extent to which you feel comfortable. If possible, involve one or both of your parents in your decision-making process. Consult with other trusted adults—relatives, clergy, doctor or counselor.

2. Learn about various adoption agencies and adoption attorneys. You may be referred by your physician or religious organization, or you may find the information in reference books. I have included several resources in Appendix B.

3. Learn about the adoption laws in your state. This is essential in order to understand your rights as a birthmother, because the laws differ from state to state.

4. Schedule an appointment with an adoption agency. Make sure that the agency is licensed and in good standing. You may also contact an attorney who specializes in private adoptions, but be sure that the attorney is reputable and has your interests at heart.

5. Discuss your various options and check on any costs involved. Ask about open versus confidential (closed) adoptions.

6. Join an adoptive parents' support group.

7. Seriously consider counseling pre- and post-adoption.

Counseling can be very valuable. It helps to be able to meet with someone who understands the adoption process and talk about your thoughts and feelings. It is essential that the counselor be trained in adoption counseling. Adoption is a challenging event, even if it is the right choice for you. With a reputable agency you will get counseling. There is no obligation to decide to place with that agency, or at all. Professional counseling is very important to help you deal with your feelings. There have been many cases of birthmothers who have not wanted counseling initially, but who have returned after a year or so for it. They were still grieving, and nobody had prepared them for those feelings.

Prior to your reaching a decision about adoption, a counselor should inform you about all your pregnancy options in a nonjudgmental way. The counselor should not tell you what to do. They should help you sort out your feelings and guide you toward making a decision. You need to know that adoption is one of your options, but that you don't need to make a final decision until after the baby is born.

Your counselor should also be able to answer the following questions:

- If I decide not to carry my baby to term, how will you help me?
- If I decide to parent rather than place my baby for adoption, how will you help me?

The counselor should discuss the various forms of adoption. The birthmother may choose to have more or less control in the adoption process. In an open adoption the birthmother can be involved in the process of selecting and meeting the adoptive parents and may maintain contact with the child. In a traditional (or closed) adoption, there is little or no contact with the adoptive parents or the child post-adoption. The counselor also needs to discuss the role of the biological father in the adoption process. Again this may vary according to state law. It may be beneficial to include your partner in the counseling.

After making a decision to choose adoption, the counselor should make sure that you are fully informed about your rights and responsibilities as a birthparent. They can help you deal with grief and loss, help you develop a support system, and discuss your future plans and goals. If you do decide to continue your pregnancy, you should be referred for appropriate prenatal care as soon as possible. Your physician may refer you to a comprehensive adolescent pregnancy program if one is available in your area.

All your options—raising your child, terminating your pregnancy and adoption—are associated with some form of loss. You have carried your pregnancy to term and you may feel emptiness after making an adoption plan. But, were you ready to marry, have a family, and be a good parent at this time? Were you ready to put in the energy and make the sacrifices necessary to raise a child? Did you have the resources (including financial) available to support a family?

If you were not ready to parent and chose to give your baby for adoption, you have made an unselfish decision and have given your baby the chance of being raised by loving adults ready and willing to parent a child at this time. In spite of knowing this, you will still grieve over your loss. Everyone grieves in their own way. Some put off their grief until later and others keep themselves very busy and try to suppress their grief. However, moving through the stages of grief is what usually will lead you to acceptance and healing.

Agency Adoptions

An agency matches the right child with the right adoptive parents. Adoption agencies may be either private or public. The private agencies can be either nonprofit or for profit. Most, however, are nonprofit organizations licensed by the state to approve prospective parents for the purpose of adoption. In an agency adoption, all adoptive parents are preapproved through an investigative process called a home study. Birthparents are usually expected to sign all final adoption papers, known as relinquishments, soon after the child is born. The child is then usually either placed in temporary foster care or with the adoptive family. Most agency adoptions are "closed," but many agencies will provide birthparents with more control by allowing them to place the baby in person with the adoptive parents of their choosing. Agencies will provide the birthparents with emotional support and counseling before and after the baby is born. They may also offer medical care and assistance with clothing and food.

The role of any agency includes responsibility to:

- Provide counseling.
- Handle legal matters.
- Make hospital arrangements for the birth.
- Select a home for your child.
- Refer you to agencies that might help you financially.

Because of their experience, agencies can expedite the adoption process, and do much of the legwork to save you time.

EVALUATING THE AGENCY

All adoption agencies are required to be licensed in the state in which they are operating. State organizations check adoption agencies on a regular basis, so call your state licensing board to check on the credentials of the agency you are considering. You should find out if it has committed any licensing violations, or if there are any major complaints against the agency.

If the agency appears to have a good reputation, ask them to send you some literature, so that you have time to study and compare agencies at home without being under pressure. After you have read about the agency, you may call to schedule an interview. You should ask them questions such as:

- How long they have been in business.
- The qualifications of the people arranging the adoptions.
- What happens if the adoption is not completed.
- Whether they arrange open adoptions.
- What type of counseling and support services they offer.
- If they will continue to offer support and counseling even after the adoption is finalized.

Independent or Private Adoptions

Instead of an agency, adoptions can be arranged through an adoption attorney. Private or independent adoption allows birthparents to choose adoptive parents on their own. You will give a "consent to adoption" directly to the adoptive parents, rather than "relinquishing" your parental rights to an agency. In both forms of adoption you do not give up your rights as a birthmother until after the birth. The baby is yours to parent until you sign your consent to give up that right. Before you sign any papers, check on whether there is a "revocation" period in your state; i.e., a time period in which you may reconsider and reclaim parental rights. There are advantages and disadvantages to both private adoptions and agency adoptions. If you are arranging a private adoption through an attorney, make sure that you check the attorney's credentials and credibility and that they are working to protect your rights.

FINDING AN ATTORNEY

The American Academy of Adoption Attorneys can refer you to an attorney who handles adoptions in your area.

Legal aid is available in most counties for people who cannot afford a private attorney.

FINDING ADOPTIVE PARENTS

Prospective adoptive parents have become more diverse. No longer are they always young or middle-aged married couples. Age limits for adoptive parents vary from agency to agency. In an adoption in which the birthparent chooses the adoptive parents, the age of the adoptive parents is determined by the preference of the birthparent.

In the case of a private or independent adoption, you will be involved in the selection of the adoptive parents.

• Personal ads: You can call the number in the ad, and get to know the prospective parents on the phone. If you want to work with the couple, have your attorney call their attorney and work out the arrangements according to what you want and the laws of your state.

• Your doctor may have a referral.
• Adoptive parents support groups.
• National matching services.
• Personal referrals through friends or family.

You wouldn't leave your child with a babysitter without checking the sitter's credentials. Neither would or should you allow your child to be adopted by someone without carefully selecting those prospective parents (or having them carefully selected by an agency if you decide to work through an agency). You want adoptive parents whom you can trust to love and parent your child well.

In almost every state, a prospective adoptive parent will be evaluated by a "home study." This is a confidential interactive process that includes both office and home visits, and the checking of references and other information. The process can take from a few weeks to several months.

Adoption Laws

If you make the decision to place your baby for adoption, you will want the process to go as smoothly as possible. Adoption laws vary from state to state. If you are married, both you and your husband must sign the adoption papers. If you are single, you must check the laws concerning fathers' rights in your area. Today, the signature of the father, if he can be found, is almost always required, before an adoption can be finalized. If the father can't be found, agencies usually try to locate him. If they are unsuccessful, the court may terminate his rights as father and after a certain period of time, the child can be released for adoption. It is important to learn about the laws in your state and how they will affect you and your baby, before making any final decisions. Read everything carefully before you sign.

Adoption Costs and Financial Support

All states allow expectant mothers to receive support for pregnancy-related expenses, although this support varies significantly from state to state. Some states only provide support for pregnancy-related health care, whereas others provide living expenses in addition to health care and other support. In an independent adoption, the adoptive parents are expected to pay for the costs of adoption, including the legal fees, medical bills, and possibly living expenses during pregnancy. It is not legal for the adoptive parents to make payments to the expectant parents that are not directly related to the pregnancy or adoption.

Financial status should not have to affect your decision regarding your pregnancy. Ask your physician, agency, attorney, or counselor to help you find information on local funding resources available to you.

Racial Equality

Sadly we have not come close to racial equality with respect to adoption. There are still a disproportionate number of couples waiting to adopt white babies, and there appears to be a racial barrier when it comes to placement of babies of other races. Many adoption agencies try to place children of color with a family where at least one of the adoptive parents is the same race as the child. However, sometimes there are not enough families waiting to adopt children of color, and so some agencies are not as welcoming to birthparents as they should be. There are some agencies, though, that specialize in finding families for children of color.

Closed vs. Open Adoptions

Before the 1970s most adoptions were what we now know as closed adoptions. Women who placed their babies for adoption had little or no say in the choice of the adoptive parents and almost never had any contact with the baby or the adoptive parents after the delivery. The reason that closed adoptions took place was to protect the privacy and reputation of the birthparent in a society where single parenthood was often viewed as shameful.

After the early 1970s, when society became more "accepting" of single motherhood, people spoke more openly about adoption, including the restrictions of closed adoptions. In the 1980s open adoptions became more available, mostly through independent or private sources. In an open adoption, the birthmother maintains personal contact with the child after adoption; that may or may not continue. This contact can be in the form of visitations, phone calls or letters. In a closed adoption, on the other hand, there is little or no contact. Many birthparents believe that by choosing an open adoption they have retained some control over their child's future and happiness, and consequently feel more at peace with their choice. It is of interest to note that open adoption has been more common in other parts of the world. I have spoken to several families from the Philippines, for example, where a woman was raising a child of her younger sister, her niece, as her own.

There is no right way for everyone, so it is important to discuss and learn as much as you can about your options in order to see what will work for you. Be careful about promises by adoptive parents (or their attorney) that you will be a third parent in your child's future. This is unrealistic.

Generally, the elements of an open adoption are as follows:

- Birthparents choose the adoptive parents.
- Birthparents and adoptive parents meet "face to face."
- Identifying information is shared.
- An ongoing relationship may be established between the child, the birthparents and the adoptive parents.

It is possible, however, to choose just how "open" an adoption will be. Talk to your counselor about the type of adoption that is best for you. Possibilities include:

- Only reading about an adoptive family and not knowing their names.
- Speaking on the telephone with them and exchanging first names.
- Meeting the family face to face.
- Staying in contact with the family and your child by visiting, calling or writing to each other.

For years open adoption met with much resistance, but it has become more acceptable as we have become aware of good results in many situations. It has its problems, but for some birthparents it has been a better alternative to closed adoption, giving them more control and peace of mind. Nonetheless, it is best to assume that you will not have long-term contact with your child who is adopted. It is not necessary for you and your grown child to have contact in order for them to be well-adjusted and mentally healthy. However, agencies or registries allow for such contacts by mutual consent, but it is a personal, individual decision that depends on your life circumstances at the time, and theirs.

SOME POSSIBLE ADVANTAGES OF OPEN ADOPTION

Supporters of open adoptions are convinced that it benefits the adoptees because it provides answers to many of the questions that they will be asking. Other arguments supporting open adoption include the following:

- If adoptees have the understanding of why their birthparents placed them for adoption, they will know that they are loved, and will not blame themselves for not being good enough.
- The adoptees will have access to what is known of their medical history.
- The adoptee can have a relationship with their birth family even as a child if they choose to do so.
- If adoptees are aware of their racial and national origins, they may have a better sense of who they are.
- The birth family can become part of the extended family.
- It may be easier for birthparents to place their child with people they have met, especially if they know they have the opportunity to be a part of their child's life.

Some Possible Disadvantages of Open Adtoption

Opponents of open adoption see it as potentially harmful to all members of the adoption triad. They believe that confidentiality is very important when it comes to adoption. They feel that:

- Exchanging pictures and letters may cause the birthparents to regret their decision.
- If the birthmother knows who the adoptive parents are and where they live, she may find them and demand her baby back.
- There will be no clear definition of who the "real" parents are.

What Research Suggests About Open Adoption

Because open adoption is relatively new in the U.S., there is not a lot of research yet about where the truth lies. The following seems to be true, though:

- Adoptive parents do not seem to fear that birthparents will intrude in their lives or demand their children back.
- Open adoptions do not appear to interfere with the sense of parenthood on the part of the adoptive parents.
- Open adoption also does not guarantee successful grief resolution.

One young woman I interviewed placed her baby with a wonderful family. They have an "open" arrangement and she sees her child on a regular basis. She sees how well her baby is being taken care of and she knows that she made the right decision. Nonetheless, she is still working through issues of grief and loss, and believes it will take some time.

Birthfathers

In the past, the birthfather was not often involved in the adoption planning. Experts say that only a very small percentage of birthfathers historically have taken an active part in adoption decision making, but some agencies report that recently, a quarter or more relinquishments have included active involvement of birthfathers. We are beginning to realize what an important role they can play in the process. One reason birthfathers don't get involved in making adoption plans for their babies is a feeling of shame at not taking responsibility to parent at the time. Sometimes a birthfather is against an adoption plan and would rather parent his child. Some birthfathers want to be more involved, but may not know how to be.

In general, birthmothers who have the support of their families and the birthfather usually do better and feel better about their decision. Of course, in certain situations this might not be possible; for example, in relationships involving violence or in cases of pregnancy resulting from rape or incest. An adoption attorney can give you information about birthfathers' rights in your state. It is not fair to say that birthfathers just don't care. Many do care deeply and may themselves need support to deal with their feelings of grief, disappointment and sometimes shame.

If You Decide on Adoption

Once you have made a decision to place your baby for adoption:

- Contact an agency or attorney if you have not already done so.
- Involve the birthfather legally—the attorney or agency can advise you on your state laws and specific situation.

• Continue your prenatal care. Eat well and exercise safely to be sure that you and your baby stay healthy.

• I strongly recommend counseling even if you feel as if you are handling your situation well. The attorney or agency should provide you with a counselor who specializes in adoption.

Even if you do decide to place your baby for adoption, you still need to make decisions such as whether you want to see, hold, or even name your baby after birth. These are your choices. Give yourself time to make them.

Cindy wanted to have as little contact with her baby as possible, so she opted for a closed adoption. She was told that holding and naming her baby would be much too traumatic for her. Many years later she wonders about whether this was true.

Sheila, on the other hand, held her baby right after the delivery, named him, and had a lot of input in choosing her baby's adoptive parents. Sheila, who became pregnant when she was 19 years old, was referred to an adoption agency, and after talking to friends and a counselor, opted for an open adoption. Her baby is now 18 months old, and to this day she can't imagine making any other choice. Still, as she speaks, I see the tears well up in her eyes. "It's easier when I visit her. When she comes to my house, I feel as if I can't let her go. She's mine! It's heartbreaking. I feel ready to parent now." It's not that she regrets her decision. Abortion would never be a consideration for Sheila and she prefers having some contact with her child, but it's still difficult. "There is no easy choice. You just have to make the best choice for you and the baby at the time—the choice you can live with." Sheila tells me she only wishes she would have waited a few years longer before becoming pregnant. She so much wants a family of her own. Sheila has matured in the past two years. She believes, as I do, that she will eventually achieve happiness and her goal of having a family, but she knows that she has much to overcome before that time.

Will My Child Wonder Why I Gave Him Up for Adoption?

As adopted children get older, they will probably start wondering about their birthparents, and will start asking more questions. Today, with adoption being less secretive, more adopted adults are realizing that their birthparents were doing the best they could under the circumstances, and that they placed them for adoption out of love. In an open adoption, you may be able to explain your feelings directly to the child, either in person or in a letter (an exchange of letters in which identities are not disclosed is allowed in closed adoptions).

I heard a beautiful true story yesterday. I was speaking to an adoptive mother who adopted a boy and a girl many years ago. They were from different families. They were closed adoptions, and there had been no contact with either of the birth families at any time. They were the happiest family and communicated well. When the children were old enough to understand, the parents told them that they had been adopted.

Then one day, when Nathan, her son, was 13 years old, the adoptive parents received a letter from his birthmother, requesting to make contact with him. They were devastated and their immediate reaction was not to tell him. Being honest people, though, they went to a minister for advice. The minister advised them to be open about the letter with Nathan, so that there would never be an issue of lack of trust in the future. It was good advice.

When they told Nathan about the letter, he jumped at the chance to meet his birthmother. He was exactly at that age when he wanted to explore and find out more about his roots. His adoptive mother broke down in tears, and she explained to Nathan that she was afraid he would leave them. Now it was Nathan who reassured her. "How could I want to leave you? You're my mom."

They arranged the meeting, and it went very smoothly. Nathan has learned that he was not rejected. He keeps in touch with his birthmother, but there is never any doubt in his mind about who his real mother is. The wonderful and unusual part of this story is that because Nathan's situation turned out so well, his adoptive mother decided to track down the birthmother of her daughter, who was 11 years old. It is now 20 years later, and they are a stable family and all remain in contact.

Rebuilding Your Life

Once you have gone through the grieving phase and have reached the stage of acceptance, it is time to start planning your future. This does not mean that you will forget about your pregnancy and baby, only that you must find peace in your own way and continue with your life—your family, your work and your education. At some point you will begin thinking about your relationships and whether marriage and children will be in your future. You will experience many different emotions and have to make many choices. Seeing a counselor and joining a birthparents' support group can help tremendously at this time.

Although it was more common generations ago for teenage mothers to place their babies for adoption, today adoption is rarely considered as a viable option. In fact, less than 4 percent of the half a million teenagers who give birth each year, place their babies for adoption. However, today adoption can be very different from what it used to be. Birthparents now have the choice of a closed or open adoption. They don't have to lose all contact with their children after adoption. Birthmothers have more control over the adoption plan for their babies. For some, it is best to separate; for others, to remain in contact with the children and the family after the adoption.

I hope that this chapter has at least given you some information you can use and an additional option to consider if you are faced with an unplanned pregnancy.

What to expect during pregnancy, labor and delivery

If you decide to continue your pregnancy, it's important for you to know what to expect at different stages of pregnancy and to take steps to ensure that you and your baby stay healthy.

In spite of the difficulties you have faced, your pregnancy can be a positive experience if you feel comfortable with your decision, and you have the support of your loved ones. Being prepared for some of the physical and emotional changes you will notice during this nine-month period can make the experience much easier.

Pregnancy is divided into three trimesters. Each trimester lasts twelve weeks. During the first trimester you will have a lot of issues to deal with. How you deal with these depends on how you feel about the pregnancy and the support you have from your partner and your family. In these first few weeks of pregnancy you may feel more tired than usual. You may also develop some nausea ("morning sickness") which usually, but not always, occurs in the morning. Your breasts enlarge and may become tender, and because your uterus also enlarges and pushes against the bladder, you will probably have to urinate more often. All these symptoms are normal. If you experience morning nausea, eating a few crackers when you wake up, then eating small meals frequently during the rest of the day may help. It's important to get enough calories and eat a variety of healthy foods during pregnancy. If you continue to feel nauseated and have trouble eating or have vomiting or dizziness, contact your doctor right away.

In the second trimester you will notice your abdomen growing larger and feel your baby moving inside you. You will probably be feeling better physically, with less tiredness and less nausea. As your pregnancy progresses, you may have difficulty finding a comfortable sleeping position, so using extra pillows—e.g., under your abdomen and between your legs—can help. Some women experience heartburn in the second trimester. If you do, eat smaller meals more often and keep away from spicy foods and caffeine.

In the third trimester you will start to notice a lot of growth in your abdomen and will feel more pressure on your bladder. You may also notice some swelling in your ankles and feet and may be more tired and a little uncomfortable, especially in the few days before you deliver. You may feel mild contractions at times. These are known as Braxton-Hicks contractions.

It's important that you see your doctor (obstetrician or other health care provider) regularly during your pregnancy to ensure that your pregnancy progresses normally and to address any concerns that you might have.

Staying Healthy During Pregnancy

Safe motherhood should really begin before pregnancy, with good nutrition, exercise, regular health care and keeping away from harmful substances, including tobacco, alcohol and illegal drugs. However, during pregnancy, it should continue, with early good prenatal care. You should watch for warning signs of problems and have them checked. Each day in the U.S., between two and three women die of pregnancy-related causes. Over half of all pregnancy-related deaths could be prevented through better access to health care, better quality of health care, and changes in health and lifestyle habits. Also, premature birth is a leading cause of problems amongst infants. This too is often preventable.

Early prenatal care can help decrease the risks of problems in both you and your baby. Women who don't have prenatal care or delay going for care are at risk of having complications that are not detected and that can lead to serious problems later. Some women don't go for early care because they don't know that they are pregnant. Others lack money, insurance, or transportation, or may not be able to get an appointment easily. Whatever the reasons, they can be overcome. Don't risk the health of yourself or your baby.

At your first visit to your doctor, you will be asked about your menstrual history, your medical and surgical history, and your obstetric history.

• Your menstrual history will help determine how far along you are in your pregnancy.

• Your medical history is important to determine whether you have any conditions that could place either you or your baby at a greater risk for pregnancy-related complications.

• Your obstetric history includes any information about any previous pregnancies or abortions.

A few lab tests will be done as needed.

If you are healthy, you will probably see your doctor about once a month for the first seven months, then every two to three weeks, then weekly. If you have any complications, or it is a high-risk pregnancy, you will need to see your doctor more often.

Pregnant teenagers need the same physical care as older pregnant women, even though they may need more emotional support because of all the difficult issues facing them. It's important, therefore, that you find a good healthcare provider or obstetrician-gynecologist (ob-gyn) with whom you feel comfortable.

How do you go about finding a board-certified ob-gyn? There are several possibilities:

• Get a referral by a relative or friend or your family doctor.
• Call your local hospital and ask for a referral.
• Check with your local health department or family planning center.

Questions to ask your physician:

• What are your office hours and do you have weekend or evening hours?
• Who will cover for you when you are unavailable?
• At which hospitals do you have privileges?
• Do you accept my insurance?
• What are your philosophies on natural births, circumcision, breast-feeding and so on?

Ongoing regular checkups are essential throughout your pregnancy, to ensure that you and the baby are doing well. Your doctor will make sure that your baby is in a good position for delivery. You will be checked for problems such as high blood pressure. Most problems are easily treatable if they are picked up early. You should contact your doctor and probably be checked right away if you develop vaginal bleeding, pain that won't go away, headaches, or dizziness. If you are unsure about any other symptoms, it's always better to call your doctor, even if all you need is reassurance.

Uncomfortable Symptoms of Pregnancy

Below are some common symptoms and some suggestions for managing them.

Nausea: During the first 12 weeks of pregnancy, some nausea in the mornings (morning sickness) is very common. It may range from mild to severe. You can try

- Eating a dry cracker or dry cereal or toast when you wake up in the morning and before getting out of bed.
- Having several small meals throughout the day, instead of two or three large ones.
- Avoiding greasy or spicy foods.

Heartburn: This is a burning feeling in your chest, caused by stomach acid splashing into the esophagus. You can try

- Eating slowly.
- Having several small meals a day.
- Not lying down right after eating.
- Sleeping on a few pillows instead of lying flat.
- Avoiding spicy foods and caffeine.

Constipation: You may find it difficult to have bowel movements. You can try

- Increasing the fiber in your diet by eating more fruits and vegetables, and whole grains such as whole-wheat bread and brown rice.
- Increasing your fluid intake.
- Doing mild exercise.

Infections in Pregnancy

Infections during pregnancy have the potential to damage the fetus. Some things to look out for:

Rubella, also known as German measles, can cause serious birth defects. You will be routinely tested for this infection during pregnancy. You are probably immune to rubella either from being exposed to the virus or from having the vaccine.

Toxoplasmosis can cause serious complications in a baby. Women can become infected by cleaning a cat's litter box, or from handling raw meat or unwashed vegetables. Frequent handwashing can help prevent this infection.

Sexually transmitted diseases, including chlamydia, gonorrhea, herpes, HIV and syphilis, among others, are a major concern, especially if you acquire them during pregnancy. They can cause serious complications in both the mother and the baby, as they can be passed from the mother's bloodstream to the baby's bloodstream and can also, in certain cases, be passed through breast milk. (See the separate section on sexually transmitted diseases.) Speak to your doctor right away if you suspect that you may have a sexually transmitted disease. If it is diagnosed early, it is usually more easily treated.

TESTING DURING PREGNANCY

A number of diagnostic tests may be done before and during pregnancy to make sure that you and your baby are healthy. They include the following:

- Test for blood type.
- Test for anemia.
- Blood glucose test for diabetes.
- Tests to screen for infections such as rubella and syphilis.
- Urine test to check for infection, diabetes or kidney problems.
- Pap smear and vaginal/cervical cultures.
- Ultrasound using sound waves to see the structures of the fetus.
- Further blood tests, amniocentesis and chorionic villus sampling (CVS) may be done, but are not routine.

GESTATIONAL DIABETES

Most pregnant women are screened, by means of a blood glucose test, for gestational diabetes ("diabetes of pregnancy"), which could cause problems in your baby if it goes untreated. This condition, which causes too high a blood sugar level, only affects 2 or 3 percent of women and happens more often in pregnant women over the age of 30, in obese women, or women with a family history of diabetes. Blood sugar levels usually return to normal after delivery.

Terminology

Here is a list of words that are useful to know when communicating with your doctor:

• *Cervix*: The lower part of the uterus (womb) with an opening connecting the uterus to the vagina. It protrudes into the vagina and allows menstrual flow to pass from the uterus into the vagina.

• *Ectopic pregnancy*: A pregnancy which grows outside the uterus, usually in one of the Fallopian tubes.

• *Embryo*: The name given to a developing human being from fertilization through the eighth week of development.

• *Endometrium*: The mucous membrane lining the inner surface of the uterus.

• *Estrogen*: Female sex hormone produced by the ovaries.

• *Fallopian tubes*: Tubes that carry the female sex cell (ovum) from the ovary to the uterus. The two Fallopian tubes are attached to either side of the uterus. The open ends of the tubes lie curled around the ovaries. After ovulation, a mature egg leaves the ovary, and travels through the fallopian tube to the uterus.

• *Fertilization*: Union of the ovum with the sperm.

• *Fetus*: An infant developing in the uterus, from the third month to birth.

• *Menstruation*: The monthly discharge of blood and cells from the lining of the uterus.

• *Ovary*: One of a pair of female reproductive glands, which hold and develop eggs and produce estrogen and progesterone. The two ovaries are situated on either side of the uterus. Each gland contains thousands of follicles or egg sacs. Once a month, in one of the ovaries, an egg matures, breaks out of its sac and travels out of the ovary. This is known as *ovulation*. When a girl is born, her ovaries contain all the eggs she will ever have, and only one ovary will release an egg each month.

• *Ovulation*: The periodic release of a mature egg from an ovary.

• *Puberty*: The period of life during which an individual becomes capable of reproduction.

• *Reproduction*: The process of conceiving children.

• *Sperm*: Mature male sex cell.

• *Uterus* (womb): The muscular reproductive organ from which women menstruate, and where a normal pregnancy develops. The uterus or womb is a pear-shaped muscular organ. Every month the lining of the uterus, known as the endometrium, thickens under the influence of hormones. If an egg is fertilized, it will become implanted in this tissue and develop into a fetus. If the egg is not fertilized, it disintegrates, and the thickened endometrial lining is shed. This monthly shedding of the endometrium is called menstruation.

• *Vagina*: The canal that forms the passageway from the uterus to the outside of the body. Sperm is released here during sexual intercourse. Menstrual flow passes from the uterus through the cervical opening and the vagina on its way out of the body.

HOW REPRODUCTION WORKS

During puberty, we notice many physical changes occurring, but other changes happen too. Most girls start having periods, and their ovaries begin to ripen eggs. Boys start producing sperm. Also, both girls and boys start having more thoughts about sex. Pregnancy can happen if only one sperm joins with one egg. Often girls are physically ready to have a baby long before they are emotionally ready to become parents. Fertilization, the joining of an egg and a sperm, is the beginning of a pregnancy.

An egg (ovum) is fertilized when it comes in contact with a male sperm cell. Millions of sperm are ejaculated into the vagina, passing through the cervix and into the uterus. They then move into the fallopian tubes, where fertilization takes place. The egg is fertilized by only one sperm cell and the rest of the sperm disintegrate. Then the fertilized egg, dividing many times on the way, moves through the fallopian tube into the uterus, where it attaches to the endometrium. When this happens, menstruation does not occur. The fertilized egg implants and begins to develop into an embryo and then a fetus. A normal pregnancy lasts about nine months from fertilization.

Taking Good Care of Yourself

Besides keeping a regular schedule of appointments with your doctor, there are many other things you can do to maintain good health in pregnancy.

HEALTHY EATING

A healthy diet is important for a healthy pregnancy. It will also make you feel better and stronger. A reasonable weight gain for a healthy pregnancy is between 25 and 35 pounds if you start off at a healthy weight. Overweight women may need to gain a little less, and underweight women may need to gain up to 40 pounds. You should check with your doctor what weight range you should aim for. In general, you will probably need about 300 calories per day more than you needed before you were pregnant. That is not the same as eating for two.

It's important to fill up on healthy foods rather than junk foods. Eat a variety of foods from the basic food groups:

1. Carbohydrates, especially the complex carbohydrates found in whole-grain cereals, breads, pasta, rice and potatoes. Whole-wheat bread and brown rice that contain whole grains are better for you than white bread and white rice. Whole grains also provide fiber, which can help prevent constipation, common in pregnancy.

2. Fruits and vegetables. These provide both vitamins and fiber.

3. Protein. If you eat meat and dairy products, you are probably getting enough. Vegetarians need to be more watchful of their diets, and make sure they are getting protein from tofu or dried beans, peas or other legumes, and whole grains, nuts or seeds.

4. Fat, which is important in the absorption of certain (fat-soluble) vitamins. We get fats from oils, meats, fish, poultry and dairy foods. It's best to limit our intake of fats, and to avoid fats in fast foods, sweets and fried foods.

If you feel like a snack, try cut-up fruits or vegetables like grapes or carrot sticks. You could make a fruit salad with your favorite fruits. My favorites are grapes, bananas, and canned mandarin oranges. Dried fruits, peanut butter, tuna sandwiches and yogurt are other good choices.

Fluids are important. Drink plenty of water every day. It's fine to drink some juice too, but best to avoid too much coffee, tea or soda.

Your doctor will probably advise you to take prenatal vitamins. Use whatever your doctor recommends. The supplements will also supply some minerals, such as calcium and iron. You can also get calcium in dairy foods like milk, cheese and yogurt, and in green leafy vegetables and sardines.

Iron is found in foods such as liver, red meat, dried beans, green leafy vegetables, dried fruits and enriched breads and cereals. Check with your physician to see if you need to take extra iron.

Folic acid, also known as folate, is a B-vitamin that can be found in some enriched foods and in vitamin pills. If women have an adequate amount of this vitamin before and during pregnancy, it can decrease the risk of having a baby with a neural tube defect (birth defect) such as spina bifida. It is now recommended that all women who could become pregnant make sure that they are getting enough folic acid every day. An easy way to be sure that you are getting enough folic acid is to take a vitamin with folic acid. Folic acid has also been added to some foods such as enriched breads, pastas, rice and cereals.

Pregnancy is not the best time to diet, unless your doctor advises you to do so. Let your doctor know if you have excessive nausea, or any vomiting, or are gaining too much or too little weight.

If you can't afford to buy the foods you need during pregnancy, you may qualify for an assistance program sponsored by the government. A social worker or the health department can help you find out if you qualify for the WIC program, for example. This is the Supplemental Food Program for Women, Infants and Children, which provides food vouchers for low-income pregnant and nursing women and young children.

EXERCISE

Exercise such as walking or swimming is fine and even beneficial during pregnancy, as long as you are healthy and have been used to exercising before pregnancy. Mild exercise, such as walking or swimming, will help you feel better and more relaxed. You will probably sleep better too. It's best not to participate in very strenuous exercises or to exercise in very hot or cold weather. Drink plenty of water before and during exercise. Do check with your doctor before starting an exercise program and do stop exercising if you feel tiredness, pain or dizziness, have trouble breathing or start to bleed.

REST

At certain times in your pregnancy, you will feel more tired than usual. In the first trimester, you may experience morning sickness, and just not want to be up and about so much. Near the end of your pregnancy, you will feel tired mostly because of the extra weight you are carrying. Make sure you get enough rest during your pregnancy.

Avoiding Harmful Substances

Smoking can cause serious harm to yourself and your baby. Babies exposed to cigarette smoke may be born too small or be born prematurely. Smoking causes, among other things, damage to the respiratory system and more frequent respiratory illnesses. It also hurts physical fitness. If you do smoke, stop if at all possible. If not, cut down on your smoking as much as you can.

No one knows how much alcohol is safe during pregnancy, so it is best not to drink alcohol at all. Babies exposed to alcohol before birth can be born with fetal alcohol syndrome. Fetal alcohol syndrome is a leading cause of birth defects and mental retardation and is preventable by not drinking alcohol during pregnancy.

Illegal drugs are very harmful to you and your baby. These drugs can cause brain damage and even death. Some babies may be born addicted. Even certain prescription drugs such as tetracycline, accutane, and some pain medications, can cause problems during pregnancy, so check with your doctor before taking any medications.

Caffeine, contained in coffee, tea, sodas and chocolate, may cause heartburn and nausea, but to date there is no convincing evidence that caffeine causes birth defects in humans. Still, many doctors recommend that pregnant women limit their intake of caffeine or avoid it altogether, because of the possible problems.

Labor and Delivery

When your contractions become stronger and closer together, or you have noticed leaking of a clear or bloody fluid, this probably means you are in labor. Most babies are born by vaginal delivery, but sometimes the doctor needs to perform a Cesarean section (C-section). If the baby is too big to come through the birth canal, or the baby isn't in a good position (e.g., a breech), or has a problem and needs to be delivered immediately, a C-section can be done. The doctor makes a cut in the mother's uterus and delivers the baby quickly.

After Delivery

Your baby will be checked by the doctor after it is born, and then quite regularly afterwards while in the hospital. A usual hospital stay for a healthy baby is about 48 hours. Not long ago, when babies were often discharged at 24 hours of age, we saw a large number of them having to be readmitted to the hospital, so now the recommended stay is about two days for a healthy baby. While in the hospital, babies' weights are checked regularly. They are also watched for signs of infection or for jaundice, which manifests itself with yellowing of the whites of the eyes and the skin. Your baby will receive a shot of vitamin K to prevent bleeding and drops or ointment will be put into their eyes to prevent infection. At birth most newborns will cry right away and then remain very alert and active for about an hour or so. This is a good time to hold and bond with your baby.

While you're in the hospital with your baby, it's an ideal time to ask any questions you might have, including questions about breast-feeding or bottle-feeding. You may also check on whether parenting classes are offered. If you have a boy and have decided to have him circumcised, this can be done within the first day or two in the hospital, or at a later date. If circumcision is done in the hospital, it is often done by the obstetrician. If your baby has any complications after birth, they can be transferred to a special care unit with highly trained doctors and nurses for further treatment.

WHAT TO PACK FOR YOUR BABY

I know this is an exciting and chaotic time, but if you forget everything else, do remember to buy a good infant car seat for your first ride home from the hospital. Other items to pack are diapers, a bottle, a pacifier, one or two newborn outfits, and a blanket for your baby, and a nightgown, a change of clothing, and cosmetics for yourself. If you do forget anything, they are well-equipped in the hospital, so don't worry. When I went into labor, my husband was so excited that he couldn't even remember the way to the hospital, let alone remember to take the bag I had packed.

WHAT TO BUY FOR HOME

• A good crib: Check to make sure that the width between the bars conforms to the safety standard and is not too large.
• Changing table (be careful of falls).
• A rocking chair (for you) is a treat.
• Infant tub.
• Baby outfits, hat.

• Infant blankets and towels.
• Bottles (even if you plan to breastfeed).
• Pacifier.
• Diapers, diaper wipes, and diaper pail.
• Nursing bras.
• Musical mobile.
• Car seat.

FEEDING YOUR BABY

Babies can thrive on both breast milk and formula. However, if you and your baby are healthy and you are undecided about bottle versus breast-feeding, I recommend breastfeeding. The American Academy of Pediatrics has recommended exclusive breastfeeding for the first six months of life and continuing breastfeeding with the addition of other foods in the next six months, as optimum nutrition regimens for infants. We continually learn about more advantages of breastfeeding for both mother and baby. The following are some of them.

1. Breast milk helps protect your baby from certain infections, including infectious diarrhea, respiratory infections and even ear infections.
2. Babies who breast-feed have less chance of milk allergy and diarrheal illness.
3. The protein, fat and carbohydrate composition in breast milk is ideal for full-term and near-term infants.
4. Breast milk is the only food your baby needs for the first six months. It is readily available and costs nothing.
5. Breastfeeding is an excellent way to bond with your baby.
6. You may lose weight more easily, as breastfeeding uses a lot of energy.

Your breast milk provides the most important nutrition for your baby's first year of life, and provides many other benefits listed above. If you decide to breastfeed, it is ideal to begin as soon as possible after delivery, preferably in the first hour when your baby is very alert. Your baby should be encouraged to feed at least 8 to 12 times a day at first. A guide to knowing if your baby is getting enough milk, is seeing about six to eight wet diapers a day. If you are having trouble nursing, speak to your doctor. Some offices have lactation consultants who deal specifically with breast-feeding issues.

Common breastfeeding problems include:

• Pain from incorrect latching and sucking.
• Pain from engorgement: This can also occur because of poor latching on. Speak to someone about how to make sure your baby latches on correctly.
• A warm shower or warm comp resses before feeding and cool compresses after feeding can also help engorgement.
• If breastfeeding is not effective, you can also be taught to express your milk (this can be done manually or, more effectively, with a pump).
• Expressed breast milk that will be used within 48 hours of collection can be refrigerated. If it will not be fed to the baby within 48 hours, it should be frozen.

An iron-fortified formula is usually recommended if you do not plan to breastfeed. Regular cow's milk is not adequate for babies before one year of age.

If you decide on bottle feeding, keep the following tips in mind:

• Read formula labels carefully.
• Follow mixing instructions properly.
• Don't put your baby to bed with a bottle of milk, juice or any sweet liquid. This can promote tooth decay.
• Don't heat the formula in the microwave.

The hospital staff and your pediatrician should be able to answer any other questions on bottlefeeding or breastfeeding.

Abortion

Legal abortion is the most commonly performed surgical procedure and one of the most controversial issues in the United States. More than one third of all pregnant teenagers choose to have an abortion. You have probably heard of two very vocal factions debating this issue. One faction known as "pro-life" opposes abortion and the other known as "pro-choice" supports the right to legal abortion. Other people, perhaps not as vocal, take the middle ground, supporting some views from each side. For example, they may agree with the right to an abortion only in cases where rape or incest occur, or if continuation of the pregnancy would endanger the life of the mother.

Since 1973, all women in the United States have the legal right to an abortion, as defined by the Supreme Court in *Roe v. Wade.* The court decided that women, in consultation with their physicians, have a constitutionally protected right to have an abortion early in pregnancy—before viability—free from government interference. If you are a minor, there may be some restrictions to this right and these vary from state to state. States can require parental notification or consent. If, for various reasons, you are unable to get consent, or do not wish to involve your parents, you can try to apply for a judicial bypass. This means that you will go to court and present your case before a judge, who will decide if you are mature enough to make your own decision to have an abortion.

In the past, making abortion illegal did not prevent its practice. Women who were determined not to carry an unwanted pregnancy always found some way to try to abort. Often, though, they resorted to dangerous and sometimes fatal methods.

In the 1950s, about a million illegal abortions were performed a year in the U.S., and over 1,000 women died each year as a result. In the 1960s, women began to fight more actively for their rights, and on January 22, 1973, the U.S. Supreme Court ruled in *Roe v. Wade* (*Marlene Gerber Fried: Our Bodies Ourselves for the New Century*. Chapter 17, Abortion). Since then, legislation has been introduced at the federal and state levels to try to regulate abortions, and these efforts will probably continue.

Abortion will always be a controversial subject and issues concerning abortion will probably always make the headlines.

Terminology

First trimester: The first 12 weeks of pregnancy.

Induced abortion: A procedure done voluntarily to end a pregnancy.

Medical abortion: Abortion brought about by taking medications that will end a pregnancy.

Miscarriage: An abortion that occurs by accident.

Surgical abortion: Ends a pregnancy by emptying the uterus with special instruments.

Therapeutic abortion: The intentional termination of a pregnancy because the pregnancy is a hazard to the mother's life and health.

Statistics

• About five million American women become pregnant each year, and almost 50 percent of those pregnancies are unintended. Half of these are terminated by abortion.

• The total number of abortions in the U.S. dropped from 1.61 million in 1990 to 1.37 million in 1996.

• Each year about 50 million abortions occur worldwide. Twenty million of these are done illegally.

• To put things into perspective as far as teenagers are concerned, 20 percent of abortions are obtained by teenagers, and two-thirds of all abortions are among never-married women (according to the Alan-Guttmacher Institute).

Why Do Women Have Abortions?

There are many different reasons why some women choose abortion.

• Sometimes a woman has an abortion because her pregnancy puts her life in danger or because her baby will suffer from serious birth defects.

• A very small percentage of women abort because their pregnancies result from rape or incest.

• Some choose abortion because of problems with their partner, concerns about single motherhood, or because of lack of money and resources needed to raise a baby.

• A woman may not want anyone to know that she is pregnant or has been sexually active.

• A woman may not want more children.

• A woman's husband, partner, or parent may want her to have an abortion.

• Most women who choose to have an abortion are young, single and pregnant for the first time. They may not feel ready to take on the responsibility of raising a child.

How did most of these young women get pregnant?:

• Some reported that they used no contraception in spite of not wanting to become pregnant.

• Some reported a contraceptive failure.

• Some were the victims of rape or incest (about one percent).

The Decision

Deciding whether to have an abortion is probably one of the most difficult decisions you will ever have to make. It is a huge responsibility. Legally you have the right to continue your pregnancy and raise your child, continue your pregnancy and place your baby for adoption, or terminate your pregnancy. Do involve your parents or another responsible adult in your decision-making process when considering abortion. However, in the end, only you can make the final decision based on your own personal, moral and religious beliefs.

Questions to ask yourself before you make the decision:

• Have I considered all the other options?

• Is this my decision or am I being pressured into making this decision?

• How does my partner feel about the decision and how does this impact me?

• How would my parents feel about the decision and how does that impact me?

• Will I still feel comfortable with my decision in the future?

If you choose to have an abortion, you may wonder if your parents need to know. Many teenagers who choose to have an abortion discuss this with at least one of their parents. However, this is only required in states with mandatory parental involvement laws. These laws require that a woman under the age of 18 (a minor), notify her parent or get permission before having an abortion. If you are a minor, your doctor or local Planned Parenthood Health Center can help you find out about the laws in your state.

Christy, a 17-year-old patient of mine and the daughter of practicing Catholic parents, came to my office crying one Friday morning. She told me that she had been pregnant and had had an abortion. She had come to the decision together with her boyfriend, who had accompanied her to the clinic where the abortion was performed. At the clinic she received minimal counseling. She had also not spoken to either of her parents, and felt she could not "live with herself" any longer. The main thing she needed was the love and acceptance of her parents. She could never hope for approval, as she knew their views on abortion.

She had not been able to find the courage to tell them up to now but did not want to keep this secret any longer. We planned on setting up a meeting in my office so that I could mediate the discussion. It took Christy two more days to consider this, but by Monday she was prepared to have a meeting. Christy, her parents and I sat down together and she slowly told them her story of her unplanned pregnancy, the abortion, and most of all about her feelings about letting them down and now needing their acceptance.

Christy was expecting the worst. I can't say that this was one of the easier discussions I've had, but her parents were more forgiving than either of us had anticipated, and although they were "shaken," it seemed as if they appreciated her honesty and were willing to provide the emotional support she needed.

When Is an Abortion Performed?

In the United States, most abortions are performed in the first trimester (first 12 weeks of pregnancy). Abortion is safest when performed during this time period. Second trimester abortions (between 12 and 24 weeks) are performed, but are more complicated. Before an abortion can be done, a medical professional must confirm that a woman is pregnant and exactly how long she has been pregnant. The length of pregnancy is usually measured by the number of days that have passed since the first day of her last menstrual period.

The longer you wait, the more difficult the procedure and the more medical complications you risk. In addition, there comes a time in your pregnancy—when the fetus is able to survive—when an abortion can no longer be performed. It is therefore important to gather as much factual information as you can, and make your decision as early as possible. Your physician will either provide information and resources, or point you in the right direction.

Since *Roe v. Wade*, women have obtained abortions earlier in pregnancy, when health risks to them are much lower. In 1973, only 38 percent of abortions were performed at or before eight weeks of pregnancy (CDC, 1974). Today, 88 percent of all legal abortions are performed within the first 12 weeks of pregnancy, and 55 percent take place within the first eight weeks (CDC, 1999).

Methods of Abortion

There are two methods of abortion: surgical and medical.

SURGICAL ABORTION

Most first trimester abortions are done by vacuum aspiration. This is a procedure done in a doctor's office or clinic, usually with local anesthesia. The contents of the uterus are evacuated through a cannula by the suction action of an electronically powered aspirator. Second trimester abortions are more complicated and various methods are used; e.g., dilation and evacuation (D & E).

Advantages of vacuum aspiration over medical abortion:

- Very effective—approximately 99 percent.
- Usually requires only one doctor's visit.
- The procedure is usually complete within minutes.
- One may be sedated during the procedure.

Disadvantages of vacuum aspiration:

- It is an invasive surgical procedure.
- It may seem less private to some women.
- It may not be readily available very early in pregnancy.

MEDICAL ABORTION

In September 2000, the United States Food and Drug Administration approved Mifepristone (RU486) for use in the United States. Mifepristone, together with a second drug, is now approved for use in early abortion. This gives American women access to a drug that has been used for many years by women in other parts of the world. This new option for early abortion could greatly reduce the number of surgical abortions done in the future.

Mifepristone was first developed during the early 1980s by researchers working for a French pharmaceutical company. The original product was refined to become the drug we now know as Mifepristone or RU486. Early studies showed that when used alone, Mifepristone induced a complete abortion in up to 80 percent of women up to 49 days' gestation. By adding a second drug a few days later, a complete medical abortion followed in nearly 100 percent of women. In 1988, France became the first country to license the combination of Mifepristone and a prostaglandin analogue for abortion during early pregnancy. Since then a number of countries have used the method for medical abortion and in September 2000, the U.S. FDA approved the use of RU486 in the U.S.

The clinical trials in the U.S. used a single oral dose of Mifepristone followed 48 hours later by a dose of oral Misoprostol. With this regimen, the highest rates of complete abortion (about 95 percent) are seen in women up to 49 days' gestation.

At her first doctor's visit the pregnant woman takes RU486 to interrupt the implantation of the fertilized egg. Two days later she take another pill, a prostaglandin, which causes contraction of the uterus, and the fetus is expelled. Two weeks later she makes a followup doctor's visit. So there are three visits in all.

Some women cannot use RU486, for example women with undiagnosed vaginal bleeding or a possible ectopic pregnancy, among other things. Side effects from the abortion process include pain and bleeding. Side effects from the medications include nausea and vomiting, diarrhea, fever and chills. Complications such as serious vaginal bleeding requiring transfusion and uterine infections are rare. About 5 percent of women will require surgery to complete the abortion.

Advantages of Mifepristone:

• Approved by the FDA for abortion.
• Usually avoids the use of surgery, so it avoids the risk of injury to the cervix or uterus.
• Anesthesia is not required.
• High success rate.
• May offer women more privacy than a surgical abortion.
• Mifepristone is given orally.
• Can be used very early in pregnancy.

Disadvantages of Mifepristone:

• Requires at least two visits.
• Not as effective after seven to nine weeks.
• Takes days or, rarely, weeks to complete.
• Bleeding after the procedure may last longer than with a surgical abortion.

Possible Complications

Prior to the legalization of abortion in 1973, many women suffered serious medical consequences, including death from illegally performed abortions. The risk in a legal abortion today is very low, but complications include problems such as bleeding, infection, and injury to the cervix or uterus. Still, the risk is one-tenth of that of carrying a pregnancy to completion. About 1.5 million American women choose to have induced surgical abortions each year. Less than one percent of all patients have a major complication associated with the procedure (National Abortion Federation).

Counseling

If you are facing an unplanned and unwanted pregnancy, you have a right to complete medical information, nonjudgmental counseling about your options, and support for whatever choice you make, whether it is parenting, adoption, or abortion. After 1973, when abortion became legal, it became standard for clinics that offer abortion services, to offer women an opportunity to discuss their options and work through their feelings about their pregnancies with trained counselors. These counselors should be able to answer questions you have about the procedure, what you should expect, and any possible complications.

Before and After an Abortion

If you do decide to go ahead with an abortion, you will need to sign a form that says:

• You have been informed about all your options.
• You have been counseled about the procedure, its risks, and how to take care of yourself afterwards.
• You have chosen abortion of your own free will.

Before you have an abortion, your health-care provider will ask you about your menstrual history, method of contraception, medical problems, surgeries, allergies, and medications you might be taking. A brief physical exam will then be done to check for any abnormalities, to determine the duration of pregnancy, and to rule out an ectopic pregnancy. A few lab tests will be performed.

Most women feel physically well very soon after an abortion. Some women, however, may have concerns about whether they will have any physical complications from the abortion, or they may have questions such as whether they will be able to get pregnant in the future. The postabortion checkup, often conducted about two weeks after the abortion to see that all is well and to make sure that there are no complications, is a good time to have the doctor answer your questions. It is also a good time to discuss future reliable contraception if you will continue to be sexually active.

Don't wait two weeks if you have serious concerns. It's important to report any severe or lasting pain, fever, or excessive bleeding to your doctor as soon as possible.

POSTABORTION CONTRACEPTION

Don't believe that because you've just had an abortion, you can't become pregnant soon. One young man I recently met thought that was true, and was devastated when his girlfriend became pregnant for the second time. Fertility returns quickly after abortion. Even within ten days, a woman can conceive again. It's very important to be aware of this, to prevent future unwanted pregnancies.

Your follow-up clinic visit is an ideal time to discuss your contraception options if you plan to be sexually active. If your unplanned pregnancy occurred while using a condom, for example, ask about factors that could have contributed to the pregnancy. Perhaps you could use the pill and a condom.

Psychological Effects of Abortion

Abortion is never easy. But it should be safe and free of pressure.

Women differ in their emotional response to an abortion. This response is influenced by whether the woman felt comfortable with her decision, her moral and religious beliefs about abortion, and whether or not she had the support of her family or her partner. Most women feel relief after an abortion and the majority continue to feel comfortable about their decisions for the rest of their lives. A small percentage of women, however, experience long-term depression after an abortion (Ava Torre-Bueno).

After an abortion, many women want to move on, and prefer not to spend much time discussing their unwanted pregnancy or their abortion. Some women do want to talk about their experience and their feelings with someone who can be caring and supportive. Talk to someone you trust. This person could be a family member, your partner, a doctor, or a counselor.

Some ways to move on and look to the future:

Some women found it helped to write down their goals in life—both short-term and long-term. Find ways to stay positive:

- Put time into studying or your career.
- Spend time on a hobby you enjoy.
- Writing, poetry or music may make you feel better.
- After having an abortion, some women find that a "letting go" ritual gives them spiritual healing.

Some Personal Stories of Abortion

Gayle's Story

Gayle was 19 years old when she became pregnant. She tells me that was the year she lost her innocence. "I never looked at the world the same way again." She had been dating Kevin for 18 months and had always believed she would marry him some day. However, although she loved him she was not ready to settle down yet. They were both still in college and Gayle envisioned a good career and a bright future. They had been in a sexual relationship for about a year and Gayle admits that they had been using contraception sporadically. When she missed a period, Gayle, who had always been "regular," had no doubt that she was pregnant. A pregnancy test confirmed this, and she knew right away what she wanted to do.

Keeping the baby was not an option for her. She wanted to complete college and she was not ready to be married, let alone have a family at the time. The idea of adoption didn't enter her mind. She knew she was going to have an abortion. Kevin was attending college out of state, so she called him on the phone to break the news. His reaction was worse than she had expected, and although he agreed with her decision about the abortion, he distanced himself from her from then on—both physically and emotionally. Gayle was in this alone. She was devastated and still feels anger towards Kevin years later.

Gayle had to speak to someone. She didn't feel as if she could go to her parents at that time (although she did months later), so she confided in her older sister, who accompanied her to the hospital clinic where she was to have the abortion. The room was cold and "sterile." Someone gave her information about the procedure, but no one counseled her or tried to change her mind. Gayle tells me the last thing she remembers while lying in her white gown and before "going under" was seeing a sign on the wall saying: "This is the first day of the rest of your life!" Gayle wasn't sure if that was a good or a bad omen.

The hardest part for Gayle was not the abortion itself, but the broken relationship and her shattered dreams. She had given herself emotionally and physically to a man who wasn't who she thought he was. She received counseling, and found this very valuable, but it was years before she dated seriously again.

After talking to many women who have had abortions, it seems that how they cope with the situation depends mostly on the support they get from their partners and their families. Gayle didn't feel she had had the support she needed and years later she still speaks about this with some hurt.

In the United States, thousands of women have abortions each day. How did they feel about their pregnancies? How did they feel about their experience? Years later, did they still suffer emotionally? Of course, each situation is unique. Much depends on your relationship with your partner, the support you receive from your partner and family, and whether you and your partner agree about having an abortion. Still, after reading the literature and speaking to many young women who have had abortions, there are many reactions and experiences that they have in common, and I will share these with you.

In the context of highly emotional situations such as abortion, it is normal to have strong feelings, such as transient depression, anxiety, or guilt (Stotland, N.L.).

Even if a woman believes in a woman's right to reproductive choice and therefore a right to choose to have an abortion, the decision can still cause her pain, guilt and grief. Although most women who choose abortion feel relief after the abortion and continue to feel comfortable with their decision years later, a small percentage do suffer from long-term depression afterward. Some women are in denial and think they are fine; then, months or years later, they are suddenly faced with difficult emotions.

Guilt is the most common negative emotion women experience after an abortion. You may feel guilty about ending your pregnancy in addition to having conceived without wanting to. Perhaps, like Gayle, you weren't using birth control regularly. You may have been using a method that was not very effective, or not using any method at all. Did you subconsciously want to get pregnant? Perhaps you were coerced into having sex, or became pregnant as a result of rape or incest. It may be important for you to look at why you became pregnant, or why you risked pregnancy at that time. Although some feelings of guilt are very common, it is difficult to move on and to heal when you continue to feel overwhelming guilt, especially when the guilt is inappropriate. Do not be afraid to ask for help if you need it. If you don't know where to go for help, your physician, a school counselor, or your local Planned Parenthood affiliate can guide you.

Another common emotion after an abortion is grief. Most women who have an abortion experience a mild feeling of sadness and loss. Even though they have chosen this path over other choices which were undesirable to them, it is still common to experience a sense of loss. We grieve when we separate from a loved one or a friend, when we lose a pet, or even when we move from one home to another. It is certainly appropriate to allow yourself to grieve in the case of abortion, even if you did make the choice. You may grieve for the lost opportunity to have that baby, or for a lost relationship, if your partner is no longer with you. You may grieve for the lack of better circumstances such as a job or more money, or for the loss of your innocence.

Gayle told me that when she looks back at her experience, what stands out most vividly is how she changed, before and after her abortion. Before she became pregnant she was a child and looked at the world through the eyes of a romantic young girl. After the abortion, she grew up fast. She was an adult now, whether she was ready or not. After an abortion, it is important to recognize your grief and work through it. In our culture it is sometimes more difficult, as it is not as acceptable to express one's grief here as it is in other cultures.

On the other hand, there are women who say that the decision to have an abortion was a turning point in their lives. Although they had to make difficult and painful decisions, they felt as if they had at last taken responsibility for their futures. It is difficult to interpret the psychological effects of abortion, and the true incidence of psychiatric illness after abortion is not known. Some women who have abortions have pre-existing psychiatric and psychosocial problems. Unwanted pregnancies occur more often in women with difficult social circumstances. Some women develop psychiatric problems or exacerbations after abortion just as they do after childbirth. In addition, women who have abortions often do not choose to have long-term follow-up, so the effects are difficult to monitor.

KAYLA'S STORY

Kayla was 19 years old when she had an abortion. She is now 30, and happily married with a three-year-old daughter. She feels as if she is a different person. "It's like looking back on someone else's life."

Kayla had been dating Pete exclusively for five years. They took their relationship pretty much for granted. Even when it came to sexual activity and discussions about preventing pregnancy, they took for granted the fact that there wouldn't be any problems. So, there really weren't any discussions, and they used condoms sporadically, and the withdrawal method when there were no condoms. Unfortunately, this system did not work, and Kayla learned that she was pregnant.

Although during the five years that they dated, Kayla fantasized about a future with him, as soon as she told Pete about her pregnancy, all illusions faded. "I knew then that he was not the one I was going to spend forever with," she said. It became obvious that he was not ready to be a father, and he had no interest in providing support in any way. When he became emotionally and verbally abusive, Kayla split up with him, and made plans to transfer to another college.

She had already made her pregnancy decision, and he was not part of the decision-making process. Kayla's parents were divorced at the time, but she felt close enough to her mother to be able to confide in her. She was shocked to find out then that her mother too had had an abortion many years before. Her mother supported her decision, and Kayla went to a clinic that provided abortion services. She took up their offer of group counseling, which helped her, and then went through the procedure without complications.

Kayla felt fine after the abortion, mostly, she believed, because she had the support of her mother. About six months later, she had some feelings of sadness, especially around young infants, and she wished she would have taken advantage of further counseling, but these feelings were short-lived. Today she is in a stable marriage, and seems to be a very good mother.

Kayla's advice to pregnant teenagers: "I have seen a number of people having second abortions for unwanted pregnancies. Don't let this happen to you. If you are going to continue to be sexually active, speak to your doctor about contraception that is more reliable. Also, if you consider abortion, counseling is so important. You need to open yourself up to finding the help you need, so that you can make the best decision."

Abortion from a Man's Point of View

A man's reaction to abortion is often overlooked. He may be feeling confused and anxious. He may also be feeling sad, guilty, afraid or even angry. The fact that he doesn't have much control over the situation makes it even harder.

Many men may not know how to deal with the situation. In the case of an unplanned pregnancy, some men have told me that they wanted to run away from the problem or deny that they were the father. Your partner, too may feel the urge to "run," still may be unsure of what to do, and may have little money. Still, he may want to take responsibility for his actions. Be open if he wants to communicate with you. Both of you should talk to your parents, another adult relative, or a counselor or health-care provider as soon as possible. You need to be informed about all your options.

Kerry's boyfriend, Steve, did not accompany her to the hospital clinic for her abortion. Kerry felt that Steve had almost no emotions at all, and their relationship deteriorated. A few weeks after the procedure, Kerry developed a high fever and had to be rushed back to hospital with a severe infection related to the abortion. This time Steve sat in the waiting room for hours waiting to hear if she would be okay. He was now filled with guilt for having contributed to her illness and was dealing with his pain for the first time after weeks of denial.

Kerry felt no sympathy for him. She felt that he now had had a taste of what she had gone through. Steve probably didn't feel as comfortable talking about his feelings. It's important to know that it is normal for men to have strong feelings too after an abortion. If you can't easily talk to and get the help you need from family and friends, do talk to a counselor or therapist.

Keeping the Secret

In an ideal situation, you would have a loving relationship with your partner and be able to discuss your plans with him and with your parents. Even if you are not required to obtain parental consent, I still encourage you to speak to them, unless you are in an abusive family situation. Some young women told me that they confided in someone else, such as a sister, an aunt, a friend, or a teacher, rather than their parents. Sometimes they would discuss the situation with their parents at a later time. Although it may be scary telling your parents that you are pregnant, the sooner you tell them, the easier it is, and usually they will be more understanding than you expect them to be. If you are afraid to talk to your parents, you can also ask your doctor or a counselor to help you discuss the situation with them.

Where Do You Begin?

1. If you think you are pregnant, find out for sure with a pregnancy test. Early diagnosis of pregnancy gives you more options. If you choose to continue your pregnancy, starting prenatal care is important to ensure a healthy outcome for you and your baby. If you choose to have an abortion, the earlier it is done, the lower the risk to you.

2. Consider all pregnancy options carefully before making your decision. A good place to start is with your own doctor or your local Planned Parenthood affiliate (call 800-230-PLAN). If you are having difficulty finding a health-care provider that performs abortions, you may also contact the National Abortion Federation.

3. Enlist the support of your family and the baby's father, if possible. Women who have this support do better later on and feel better about the choices they made. If you are unable to involve your family, try to find the support of another responsible adult.

4. Schedule an appointment with a health-care provider as soon as possible.

5. Get as much information as possible about all options available to you. Learn about your legal rights.

6. If you opt for abortion, check your state laws regarding parental notification and parental consent. These laws vary from state to state.

7. Get preabortion counseling.

8. Obtain a list of resources available to you in your area.

Ways to Prevent Abortion

1. Preventing unwanted pregnancies through abstinence.

2. For those young people who are sexually active, increasing knowledge about and access to contraception.

Millions of Americans either do not have access to contraceptives, or don't know how to use them properly. Others may not have the money to buy them. For some teenagers, a language barrier may prevent them from having sufficient knowledge about contraception.

Since the early 1970s, Title X, the national family planning program, has established thousands of community family planning centers, and has served millions of low-income women and teenagers. By preventing unplanned pregnancies, these programs help prevent hundreds of thousands of abortions. Not everyone embraces these family planning services, however.

Young people get a lot of their information and misinformation from movies, television and their peers. Parents and teachers need to educate them about sexuality, reproduction, responsibility and consequences. They need to be given all the facts in order to make their choices. Giving them information about sexuality, abstinence, and contraception, does not increase promiscuity. I believe that teenagers will make better choices if they have a comprehensive understanding of the facts. Sexuality education programs should also help teenagers understand that waiting until one is ready to have sex is a legitimate and wise option. You as teenagers should expect this type of education.

3. For pregnant teenagers, providing education about other options— parenting and adoption.

Don't forget the fathers!

In past generations, teenage mothers often tried to do "the right thing" by marrying the baby's father. Today, with less stigma attached to single parents and with younger teenage mothers, this is not always the case. Unfortunately, even if teens do marry, the teenage divorce rate is very high. Just as being a very young mother is associated with difficulties, being a teen dad is very stressful too. Early fatherhood interferes with finishing school. Young dads are less likely to receive high school diplomas or more likely to complete high school at a later age. They therefore have more difficulty finding satisfying well-paying jobs. Teen dads also experience a loss of their freedom, change in their relationships with friends, and a higher incidence of anxiety and depression. One dad I spoke to has virtually stopped going out with his friends. He finds he has less in common with them now that he has a daughter, and believes he will have enough time to socialize when she gets older.

Millions of children grow up with no father in the home, while millions more have a dad in the home who is not emotionally involved in his child's life. However, although the teenage divorce rate, the absence of young fathers, and nonpayment of child support are major problems in our society, there are many instances where young fathers do take responsibility and stay involved in the lives of their partners and children. One study showed that two-thirds of African-American teenage fathers saw their 18-month-old infants at least three times per week (Yogman & Kindlon, *Pediatric Annals*, Jan. 1998. Ref. to Rivera et al., *Pediatrics*, 1986). Some fathers care very much, but don't know how to be supportive and how best to be involved, so teenage parenting programs exploring ways to engage young fathers in the lives of their children have now been created.

Teenage fathers are less likely to marry the mother of their children than are older men. It is important to establish legal paternity. Even if the father does not actively participate in his new family's life, he is still responsible for child support until his child is 18 years of age. Fathers can be involved in their children's lives on many levels, including being direct caregivers, teaching, arranging childcare or providing financial support, and many unmarried teenage dads do provide at least some of the above.

The Benefits of an Involved Father

Fathers play a very important role in the development of infants and children. These days dads are expected to be much more involved than just providing money. The father is a role model, a teacher and a disciplinarian. He lays the foundation for the physical, emotional and psychological development of his children. Boys watch their fathers, identify with them, and try to behave like them. Fathers even play with their children differently than mothers do, and both kinds of stimulation are important to a child's development. When fathers do put in the time and the energy, they usually find that there are great rewards.

Not having an involved father can put a child at risk for behavioral problems, academic problems, and poverty. On the other hand, the positive effects of a father's involvement can be seen even in the first year of life (Yogman & Kindlon, *Pediatric Annals*, Jan. 1998). Hospitals are therefore encouraging the presence of fathers during labor and delivery, and hospital personnel are including fathers in the instruction on feeding, bathing and changing their babies. This early involvement seems to help with bonding between father and baby. The presence and support of the baby's father can also help lessen the mother's distress at this time. It goes without saying that the father needs to be loving and caring, and sensitive to the needs of his child, rather than indifferent. Even in situations where the child is living primarily with the mother, if the father is caring, it is beneficial to allow him to keep in contact with his child as often as possible, in person or by phone.

John and Rina don't get along at all. Unfortunately, they only realized that after they had a son together. Together they made the decision to continue the pregnancy when they thought there was a chance that things would work out between them. They never married and, when the arguing became too intense, they broke off their relationship. Their baby Justin was only a year old. John lives in an apartment on his own now, and Rina and Justin have moved in with her parents temporarily.

Although John and Rina are not on friendly terms, she admits that he is a good father to his son. He spends time with him every week, takes him for walks, and reads to him. Rina has wisely decided not to interfere with that bond.

The relationship seems to be good for Justin, and John helps her out by spending those days with him, so that she can have a break. They both date other partners casually, but neither is involved in a serious relationship.

I have not found this situation happening with many couples who have separated. In spite of knowing the benefits of having two involved and caring parents, it's difficult to achieve this when the parents are fighting. If you are in this type of situation, with a partner who would like to be involved, try to encourage his involvement for the sake of your child.

Fathers Involved in Pregnancy and Childbirth

Many years ago it was almost unheard of for a father to attend prenatal visits, let alone be present in the delivery room for the birth of his baby. Now this is becoming more common, and often expected of him. Many men feel awkward, especially if they haven't been very involved during the pregnancy. They often don't know what is expected of them, and may even feel as if they are getting in the way.

For most couples, when fathers do get involved, it often helps both relax and feel more secure.

How can a father become more involved during the pregnancy?:

• Nothing can substitute for a loving, caring relationship.
• A man can go with his partner to some of her prenatal checkups, and he should feel free to ask questions. Maybe he could listen to the baby's heartbeat or see the baby on an ultrasound.
• He can read about pregnancy and what to expect during labor and childbirth.
• He can go with his partner to childbirth preparation classes.
• He can be present in the delivery room if allowed and if his partner feels comfortable with this.
• He can help plan for the baby's arrival.

• He can share his feelings with his partner. Both partners may be feeling anxious, and good communication can help.

How can a father become more involved after his child is born?:

• If he is not living with the mother of his child, he can try to live close to where the child lives, so that he will be able to see the child more frequently and not have to deal with long commutes.
• He can read about fatherhood. Although there are not as many resources for single fathers as there are for mothers, parenting magazines and websites for teen dads do exist.
• He can go to the child's pediatrician visits whenever possible. This is an ideal time to ask questions and to feel part of a child's development.
• He can consider joining a teen dads' support group.
• He can find out about activities that he can do with his child.
• He can be a good role model.
• He can ask for help. Parents or another family member may offer support. Help is also available from doctors, counselors, and members of the clergy.
• He can try to enjoy his role as father. Men, remember: You can't change the past, but you can try to make good decisions for yourself and your child from now on.

Too often teenage dads are unwillingly excluded from their child's life. For fathers who want to be involved, it doesn't have to be this way. Even young fathers can find that developing and maintaining a strong relationship with their child can be very rewarding.

Not enough is written about teenage fathers, and therefore I met with and interviewed several dads to get their side of the story.

RICK

Rick and his girlfriend were both 18 years old when she became pregnant. "It was a complete shock," Rick told me, "especially as we were using birth control." They both knew that they were not ready to parent a child, and neither was comfortable with the prospect of an abortion, for moral and religious reasons. It just so happened that a family friend was waiting to adopt a child. This seemed like their best option, and arrangements were made quickly. Even though Rick knows where his baby lives and who the adoptive parents are, he does not keep in contact with her. "I don't want to interfere in her life. I don't want her to be confused. When she's older, if she decides to come for me, I'll be here for her." I asked Rick if he had any advice for teenagers. "We could never believe this could happen to us. It can happen to you too. Don't take chances."

MARCUS

Marcus was 19 when his girlfriend Tasha became pregnant. They had dated for two years but had never considered marriage or children, so her pregnancy was very unexpected. After counseling, they decided that Tasha would have the baby and they would parent their child together, but soon after their son was born, they split up. Marcus wants to be involved in his child's life, but has to be satisfied with occasional weekend visitations. "I love my kid so much. I try and I try, but she hardly ever lets me see him." Marcus tries to do the right thing. He pays his monthly child support payments. He has joined a program to help him get a job, and attends classes to further his education. "I feel as if Tasha and I could still be friends for the sake of our child, but she doesn't want to," says Marcus. "There's nothing like when you love your child so much and you can't be with him." Marcus spoke to me for a long time. I could hear the pain in his voice and I asked him how he would advise other young men going into relationships. He answered passionately: "You need to be ready to parent—emotionally and financially. Wait till you're ready! If you do have sex, use protection. It's no joke." As I left he added: "It's not easy by a long shot, but I don't want my kid to grow up and ask me why I ran out on him, so I have to be here for him. For the rest of my life, he'll always be my kid."

ROBERT

Robert's story has a happier ending. He had dated his 17-year-old girlfriend, Celia, on and off for a few years. He says that most of their problems related to her living with her mother. Robert himself was only 18, so when Celia became pregnant, he was unprepared. However, they both decided that they were going to stay together. Robert joined a young fathers' support group and managed to get a reasonably well-paying job. They then both had incomes and were able to move into their own apartment. They continued to stay in touch with Celia's mother, with whom they have a good relationship now. When I met them they had just married. They understand that the road ahead will be tough, but with their willingness to make things work and with a good support system, they have confidence in their future together.

RAMI

I recently met 24-year-old Rami. Rami has a five-year-old daughter who moves between his home and her mother's home. She ends up spending one week night and every other weekend with her dad. Rami had been dating Amy for about a year when she became pregnant at the age of 19.

How could it happen? This is the question Rami still asks himself. Amy had been ill for a while and had required "some sort of" surgical procedure. They both thought that she would not become pregnant, so, although they were sexually active, they used no contraception. Rami was shocked when he learned that she was pregnant. He had not considered marriage in his near future. When I asked about Amy's feelings, he said that he believed that she thought this would bring them closer together.

What made things more complicated was that Amy and Rami were from two very different cultures. They knew that their families would be devastated, so they waited as long as possible before confiding in them. Rami told me he did not speak to anyone about the pregnancy until his daughter was born.

For Amy this wasn't an issue. Although she and Rami were going to split up, she wanted to continue her pregnancy and parent her baby. Rami told me he would have opted for an abortion, but went along with Amy's decision.

Rami's advice now: "Use contraception! It sounds so obvious, but no-one listens. They don't believe it can happen to them. And believe me, it changed my whole life."

Rami is a good dad. He sees his daughter as often as is allowed, and wishes he could spend more time with her. He carries a photograph of her with him wherever he goes, and when he showed it to me, I could see the pride in his face and the tears in his eyes.

How has this changed his life? Well, Rami spends very little time hanging out with his friends or seeing movies as he used to love to do. He doesn't date at this time, as he wants to devote all his spare time to his daughter while she is young. He also struggles a little financially, but pays regular child support, and is able to manage.

STEVE

We often hear about the single mother with young children, who eventually starts dating. She looks for a man who will interact well with her children, and is willing to accept them, because her children come first.

Steve's situation is reversed. He is a young man, a single father, with two little children in his custody. His girlfriend had become pregnant at the age of 17, and then again at 18. They married as soon as they were able, and Steve hoped to have a stable life. Unfortunately, his wife, Cindy, developed a drinking problem, which escalated to such a point that they divorced after two years and a judge awarded Steve custody of his children for the time being.

Steve deals with much the same issues as a single mom would, although it is a little harder for Steve, as he doesn't have as many resources available to him, and he doesn't have a large "single dad support group" with whom he can share ideas and experiences. "Only in the movies do we see the young single dads all hanging out at the park together. Maybe one day!" he says. He does have a small business that he operates out of his home, and he does have an occasional babysitter who comes in on the days that he has to work outside the house.

He is one of the most caring dads I have met, and hopefully he will find a wonderful relationship for himself one day. For now, he dates occasionally, but won't let that interfere with his time with his kids.

Prevention and contraception

Too few teenagers get regular preventive health care. They either lack access to care or seek it only when they become ill. Regular checkups during the teenage years can prevent and identify many medical and social problems seen in adolescence.

There are many reasons to discuss pregnancy prevention. The United States has the highest teenage pregnancy rate of all developed countries. Even though the rate dropped in the nineties, the numbers are still staggering. Just under one million teenagers become pregnant each year. More than three-quarters of teenage pregnancies are unintended, and almost one-third end in abortions.

Teenagers are also at high risk for sexually transmitted diseases. We see the highest rates of gonorrhea, chlamydia and human papillomavirus (HPV) in adolescents. These are only a few of the sexually transmitted diseases we worry about. AIDS is now the sixth leading cause of death among 15- to 24-year-olds.

A number of factors can increase your risk for an STD, including early onset of sexual activity and multiple sexual partners. If you have any of the symptoms such as vaginal discharge or itching, frequency of or burning on urination, fever, or abdominal pain, it's important to be tested as soon as possible. If you are sexually active, I also recommend that you be tested even if you have no symptoms, as it is not unusual for women to have infections such as chlamydia with no symptoms at all. If you are diagnosed with a sexually transmitted disease, it is important to have any sexual partner tested, and treated if necessary, to prevent the spread of infection or any reinfection.

Another reason to focus on prevention is to save society billions of dollars. Public costs from teenage childbearing totaled $120 billion between 1985 and 1990. Forty-eight billion dollars could have been saved if each birth had been postponed till the mother was at least 20 years old (CDC).

You may wonder why I put a chapter on preventing pregnancy in a book written for pregnant teenagers. Isn't it too late to be talking about preventing a pregnancy? It's never too late. A significant number of teenagers who have an unplanned pregnancy will later have second and even third unplanned, unwanted pregnancies. About one in five births to teenagers is a repeat birth (The Guttmacher Report on Public Policy—Vol. 3, no. 3, 6/2000).

Carrie was 16 years old when I met her and was pregnant for the second time. Although Carrie had not wanted either pregnancy, she admitted that she had not used contraception. After her first pregnancy she had intended to start using birth control pills, but "never got around to it." In the heat of the moment it may seem unromantic to think about birth control. Believe me, though, it's a lot more romantic to plan and care, than to have a moment of passion followed by an unwanted pregnancy and all its consequences.

One teenager told me she didn't believe she could get pregnant "the first time." Wrong! She could and did. Many women also wrongly believe that they can't get pregnant while breastfeeding or until they've had a period. When you get your period it means ovulation took place two weeks before.

Even though it is encouraging to see that the number of sexually active teenagers using contraception has increased (mostly due to increased use of condoms), they may still use contraception incorrectly or irregularly. Most unintended pregnancies among contraceptive users occur because of inconsistent or incorrect use (A.G.I. Facts in Brief. Contraceptive Use, 1998). But no matter what form of contraception you do use, remember that nothing works 100 percent of the time—nothing, that is, except abstinence.

Abstinence

The safest way to avoid pregnancy and infection is not to engage in sexual activity at all. Continuous abstinence means abstaining from having any sex play with a partner. Some people practice periodic abstinence, where they abstain from intercourse on the days they think they could become pregnant. This is not reliable.

Continuous abstinence is 100 percent effective in preventing pregnancy, and also prevents sexually transmitted diseases. Sexual relationships pose physical and emotional risks, especially to teenagers. Abstinence helps you postpone taking those risks until you are physically and emotionally ready. Women who abstain until their twenties, and who have fewer partners in their lifetimes, are less likely to get sexually transmitted infections, become infertile, or develop cancer of the cervix. Nearly 20 percent of young people do not have sexual intercourse during their teenage years (SIECUS).

Young men and women choose abstinence for a number of reasons:

• Having sex before marriage would be against their religious or moral beliefs. Most religions have strong views on sex before marriage.
• Not being ready emotionally for a sexual relationship. You don't have to give reasons. If it doesn't seem right, wait.
• Fear of an unwanted pregnancy.
• Fear of a sexually transmitted disease.
• Not having met the appropriate partner.
• Getting over a breakup.
• Wanting to keep a more friendly relationship without the pressure of sexual involvement.
• Being busy with career, schooling, or other activities.
• Illness.
• Distance from one's partner.
• Relationship problems.

Having sex before you are ready can leave you with long-term feelings of hurt, frustration and disappointment. Do wait until you have a loving committed relationship.

Charlene is 18 years old, and a college freshman. She is an outstanding student, popular with male and female friends, and full of confidence. She was proud to tell me that she was not sexually experienced. She has a steady boyfriend, but does not feel the time is right. She feels no need to discuss this with her friends, and no need to make excuses. She believes she'll know when she is ready and will not be pressured into having sex until that time. Her boyfriend respects her for this, and neither loves the other any less.

Relationships and Dating

An important element in any relationship, be it with a boyfriend or girlfriend, a family member or a friend, is respect. You must have respect for the other person and respect for yourself. Everyone has self-worth, and should be treated with dignity. Everyone is entitled to their own feelings and morals. You should not be made to do something you don't want to do. In turn, it is important that you treat others fairly, as you would have them treat you.

Couples in healthy relationships trust each other and can communicate openly. This trust and respect also relates to sexual behavior. If a partner says no, they mean no. Partners should not pressure each other to go against their values. In a healthy relationship, sexual decisions should be made together, in a responsible way.

Sadly, not all relationships are healthy. Sexual abuse does occur. Although this may be very difficult to talk about, if you have been sexually abused, you must talk about it to a trusted parent, friend, teacher, counselor, or clergy member, who may be able to help. For more information, call the National Child Abuse Hotline at 1-800-422-4453.

A sexual relationship can be a positive experience when it is based on mature, informed and responsible decisions, and in the context of a loving committed relationship.

You should be able to

- Choose when you are ready to have sex.
- Choose your partner carefully.
- Choose what you do and don't want to do with your partner and when.
- Choose to do it in the safest way.

If you have decided to have sex, ask yourself the reasons:

- Is it curiosity?
- Are you being pressured into having sex?
- Do you think that having sex will make you feel better about yourself or more sexy?
- Do you think your partner will love you more if you sleep with him?
- Are you lacking support at home and do you believe that you can only find intimacy and affection this way?
- Do you think that "everyone else does it?" Actually, many teenagers think that their peers are more sexually active than they really are.

Sexuality is normal and healthy, but don't have sex for the wrong reasons!

HOW DO YOU KNOW IF YOU ARE IN LOVE?

Can you believe that I asked myself this question one month before I met my husband. I was dating somebody and wasn't sure whether he was "the one." I was introduced to my future husband soon after, and after we started dating for a while and got to know each other very well, it became clear what love was. I still don't think I could answer this question for anyone else, though.

People have different ideas of what it means to be in love. Infatuation is an intense, exciting, "giddy" kind of feeling. When you are infatuated with somebody, it's hard to think of anything else or anybody else. Infatuation is often mistaken for love, but it usually doesn't last long, whereas true love does.

You don't have to know someone very well to be infatuated with that person. True love takes more time. You have to know someone's good and bad qualities. If you still decide you care and you want to stay together, there is a good chance it might be love. Love is a more secure, safer feeling, based on trust, companionship, and respect.

Laura was 15 years old and had dated Brad for seven months. She was happy with their friendship and enjoyed going out with him, but did not feel ready for a sexual relationship. Brad, on the other hand, believed that he was ready for one and had tried to pressure Laura into having sex with him several times. Finally, Laura, believing that she would "lose him" if she didn't sleep with him, gave in. In fact, sleeping together did not strengthen their relationship and they broke up about a month later when Brad became bored. It took a long time for Laura to get over the experience, she said. "I felt cheap and used. That's not the way I imagined sex would be the first time."

This is not an easy time to be a teenager. You may be faced with pressures from friends. If you are a high school senior, a number of your peers are probably sexually active. You are also bombarded with sexual messages on television, the internet and in magazines. Then there is the added threat of an increasing number of sexually transmitted diseases, including AIDS. Who do you talk to? Whose values do you adopt? Hopefully you have parents who can listen to you and guide you. Hopefully you won't be pressured into having sex with someone you don't love, as Laura was. Laura now knows that there is a big difference between love and sex. Also, consider this: many sexually experienced teenagers say that if they had to do it over again, they'd wait a little longer before having sex for the first time.

The Importance of Education

Abstinence outside of marriage is ideal, but two-thirds of American 12th graders are sexually active, so education about contraception, pregnancy and sexually transmitted diseases is essential. A recent study indicated that many students in secondary public schools are not receiving accurate and adequate information on topics such as birth control (Darroch, et al).

How can I impress upon you the fact that it can happen to you. If you are having sex, you too can become pregnant or contract a sexually transmitted disease or both. When I was writing this book, I was thinking about how I could stress the importance of abstinence, or contraception, if you are sexually active. Then I met Jeane! How do I even begin telling you about Jeane? Jeane S. Stockheim is one of the liveliest, most intelligent and fun-loving women I've ever met. She loves shopping, jewelry and clothes. She also has a serious side, though. She has been in the health-care field for many years and is a passionate advocate for practicing safer sex. She made me blush when I saw her collection of condom earrings and necklaces. "Always be prepared," she says.

I always think about Jeane when I talk about prevention, and I always hope I'll be as energetic when I get to be her age. Jeane, the collector of condom earrings, is 87 years old!

In life there are so many events we can't prevent. However, sexually transmitted diseases, AIDS, and unwanted pregnancies can be prevented. Think about it and do something about it.

Contraception

Studies show that teaching teenagers about contraception does not make them more likely to have sex, although I've heard people say that it does. In order to prevent the risk of pregnancy and sexually transmitted diseases completely, nothing is as effective as abstinence. However, if you have decided to have sex, and you don't want to become pregnant, you must use contraception. Vaginal intercourse without birth control, even the first time, can cause pregnancy and sexually transmitted diseases. No method of birth control is 100 percent reliable, but it can certainly make you worry less about an unwanted pregnancy than if you don't use any method at all.

I have interviewed many teenagers for this book, and they have been the ones to come up with some of the best advice.

Ron said: "Don't think it won't happen to you. I did, and I am now a single dad."

Sarah said: "Spontaneity is not all it's said to be. Life is not like a TV soap opera, where no one talks about contraception. In real life, if you don't use contraception, you can get pregnant and you can get AIDS."

Tammy was shocked that she became pregnant. "We didn't use contraception, because we didn't plan to do it. It just happened!" Sex doesn't just happen. You make the conscious decision to have sex, and it's up to you to delay that decision until you are ready.

Once you have decided to have sex, you must decide on a method of contraception. Your contraceptive needs can change throughout your life and even through your adolescence. Decide what method is best for you now.

How do you choose the best form of contraception for you? Consider the following:

- Safety.
- Effectiveness.
- Will you be able to comply?
- Will it fit your lifestyle?
- Is it affordable?
- Is the method reversible?
- Does it prevent sexually transmitted diseases?
- What are the side effects?

The contraceptive method teenage women most frequently use is the pill, but with concerns about sexually transmitted diseases, especially AIDS, the condom is also popular. Condoms are most frequently used for first-time sexual experiences.

ORAL CONTRACEPTIVES ("THE PILL")

Oral contraceptives, first developed in the 1960s, are pills containing the hormones estrogen or progestin or a combination of them. The pill works in part by inhibiting ovulation. It also causes the cervix to produce a thicker mucus (which sperm can't easily penetrate) and keeps the lining of the uterus thin to prevent the egg from implanting. Even though there has been much negative publicity associated with the pill, it is still considered safe for most young women. The highest risks are seen in smokers and women over the age of 35 years. There are a number of pills on the market. Speak to your clinician about finding the right pill for you.

Advantages of oral contraceptives (lower dose formulations):

• Very effective when used properly. Women who take the pill consistently and correctly have less than a one in a hundred chance of becoming pregnant.
• Generally safe (check contraindications and precautions with your doctor).
• Decreases the risk of ovarian and uterine cancer.
• Easily reversible.
• Reduces the risk of fibrocystic breast disease and cystic ovarian disease.
• Regulates menstrual periods.
• Lessens painful periods.
• Some pills help control acne.
• Nothing to insert before intercourse.

Side effects of oral contraceptives:

• Nausea, breast tenderness, fluid retention, and weight gain may be experienced, although less often with the newer oral contraceptives.
• Some women may notice breakthrough bleeding (bleeding between periods), headache, or acne; however, all these side effects are usually easily manageable.
• For many women, the side effects are limited to the first few months, while the body adjusts to the hormones; then they disappear.
• Serious side effects, including stroke, high blood pressure, and blood clots, are rare in teenagers. The incidence increases in smokers and women over the age of 35.

Many teenagers worry that the pill with cause weight gain. Although some women gain weight while using the pill, others lose weight. Hormones in the pill may cause changes in appetite. These changes can cause weight loss or gain. Some women gain weight due to temporary fluid retention during the first month or two after starting the pill, and some gain weight as a side effect of estrogen use. With the lower dose formulations used today, both side effects and weight gain are less common.

If the pill is so effective, why do some women who take the pill become pregnant?

- They don't take the pill correctly.
- They don't take the pill every day.
- They stop using the pill after some time and do not use another method.
- They don't take the pills in the correct order.

Why do some teenagers use contraceptives incorrectly or ineffectively? It could be they fit into one of these categories (do you?):

1. Some teenagers believe that a pregnancy could never "happen" to them. They deny the fact that they could become pregnant or cause a pregnancy.

2. Incorrect facts: Some believe wrongly that if they have sex only during a certain time of the month, they won't become pregnant. This is not reliable.

3. Spontaneity: "It just happened." Some may not have prepared for sexual activity, or they might have believed that planning or using contraception would detract from the spontaneity or romance. When an unwanted pregnancy or sexually transmitted disease occurs, the spontaneity no longer seems romantic.

4. Some adolescents want to become pregnant. They may believe that a pregnancy will improve their relationship or ensure that their partner stays with them forever, or they may want a baby who will love them and whom they can love.

5. Lack of knowledge about contraception: Some teenagers may want to use contraception, but may not have all the facts, may be concerned about certain side effects, or may not know how or where to obtain contraception.

6. Some may stop the pill, for example, because of side effects, and not use any contraception at all, instead of speaking to a health-care provider about switching to a different pill or to a different method.

7. They may have difficulty complying with daily use of the pill.

8. They may worry that their parents will find out that they are taking the pill.

Ideally before starting the pill you should have a visit with your doctor or health-care provider. At this visit a complete medical and sexual history will be taken, and a physical assessment, including weight and blood pressure, will be made. The pelvic exam, which might involve a pap smear, will exclude any gynecological problems.

The following are lab tests that are sometimes done (only when indicated) before prescribing the pill:

- Blood tests, including blood count, liver function, cholesterol.
- Urine test.
- Pregnancy test.
- Screening tests for sexually transmitted diseases.

Most doctors schedule a follow-up visit for patients about a month after starting them on the pill, to monitor weight and blood pressure and to discuss any questions they might have. It is up to you to call your doctor if you have any concerns before that time, or you develop symptoms such as abnormal (breakthrough) bleeding, abdominal pain, severe leg pains, or headaches.

You will take one pill a day, one pack of pills per month, as directed by your physician or health-care provider. The pill, if taken regularly and correctly, is very effective (more than 95 percent) in preventing pregnancy. It does not, however, prevent the transmission of sexually transmitted diseases. Use a condom in addition to the oral contraceptive to increase your protection. Oral contraceptives should be taken at the same time each day to keep levels of hormones constant and to increase their efficacy. The pill is obtained by prescription from your doctor or a clinic. In most cases an examination is required before starting the pill.

Remember:

- Take your pill at the same time each day.
- Schedule it at the same time you do another daily routine like brushing your teeth.
- If you forget to take a pill, take it as soon as you remember. It's best to let your doctor know that you've taken one late.
- Don't smoke if you're taking the pill. It can increase your risk of blood clots, stroke and heart attack. (In general, women over the age of 35 and smokers are at higher risk.)
- Antibiotics and some other medications may decrease the effectiveness of the pill, so check with your doctor if you are taking any medications.

CONDOMS

Condoms are the contraceptive method most often used during first intercourse and among younger sexually experienced teenagers.

A latex condom is a relatively good contraceptive when used correctly, and also helps to prevent the transmission of sexually transmitted diseases. For the male using the condom, it provides a mechanical barrier that should decrease the risk of infection acquired through exposure to infectious genital secretions and lesions. Proper use of the condom should also protect his partner from contact with urethral discharge, exposure to lesions on the head of the penis, and deposition of semen. However, condoms are not 100 percent effective in preventing the spread of infection. For infections spread from lesions rather than fluid, condoms may not be as protective, as the condom may not cover all infectious areas of skin. When condoms do fail to protect against sexually transmitted infections, though, it is probably more likely due to incorrect use of the condom, rather than product failure.

Recommendations for proper use of condoms to reduce the transmission of STDs:

- It is essential that you follow the instructions correctly.
- A new condom needs to be used every time you have sex.
- Condoms need to be stored properly. Store them in a cool, dry place out of direct sunlight.
- Don't use condoms in damaged packages or those that show obvious signs of age.
- Handle condoms carefully to prevent breakage or puncture.
- Latex condoms are preferable to natural membrane condoms ("skins") because they offer greater protection against viral STDs.

The condom is believed to be about 88 percent effective. Efficacy is increased if it is used with perfect technique and together with spermicidal foam or the pill.

Remember that even though condoms lessen the risk of sexually transmitted diseases, there is no such thing as "safe sex." If you are unsure of your partner's sexual history, it's better to have no sex at all.

Advantages of condoms:

- Cheap and easily available.
- No prescription is needed.
- Few side effects.
- Offers some protection against sexually transmitted diseases.
- Offers some protection against cervical cancer.
- Allows men to take some responsibility for birth control.

Disadvantages and side effects of condoms:

* Allergy to rubber in the condom.
* Allergy to nonoxynol–9 used in spermicide.
* Decreased sensation.
* Need to use with each act of intercourse.
* Possible breakage.

NORPLANT AND DEPO-PROVERA

Norplant is a long-acting hormone that is implanted under the skin in capsule form by a clinician. Its active ingredient is progestin, which prevents the release of an egg and thickens cervical mucus so that the sperm does not join the egg.

Advantages of Norplant:

* It is more than 99 percent effective.
* It protects against pregnancy for about five years.
* You won't need to take a daily pill.
* There is nothing to insert before intercourse.
* It can be used by some women who can't take the pill.

Disadvantages and possible side effects of Norplant:

* Norplant is not effective against sexually transmitted diseases. A condom should also be used.
* Side effects can include irregular bleeding, weight gain, headaches, nausea, acne, and depression.
* Some women develop scarring or infection at the incision site. This is unusual, though.
* Pregnancies, which rarely occur, are more likely to be ectopic.

Depo-Provera also contains the hormone progestin. It is given by injection by your health-care provider every 12 weeks.

It works by preventing the release of the egg, thickening the cervical mucus to keep sperm from joining the egg, and preventing the fertilized egg from implanting into the uterus.

Advantages of Depo-Provera:

* You don't need to remember to take a pill each day.
* Like Norplant, it is more than 99 percent effective in preventing pregnancy.

- It protects against pregnancy for 12 weeks.
- It decreases menstrual cramps in some women.
- It can be used by some women who can't take the pill.
- You don't have to carry a pack of pills, so it is a more private form of contraception.

Disadvantages and possible side effects of Depo-Provera:

- It does not protect against sexually transmitted diseases. Use a condom in addition to this method.
- Side effects may include irregular bleeding or absence of periods, headaches, depression, weight changes, or abdominal pain.
- Pregnancies, which rarely occur, are more likely to be ectopic.
- May be associated with some bone mineral loss.

DIAPHRAGM AND CERVICAL CAP

The diaphragm and cervical cap are not the usual contraceptives of choice for teenagers, but they are reasonable alternatives if neither the pill nor the condom is an option. The cup-shaped "diaphragm" is inserted into the vagina to cover the cervix and the surrounding area. The smaller rubber cervical "cap" is also inserted into the vagina and fits snugly over the cervix. Both methods provide a barrier between the sperm and the egg and should be used with a contraceptive jelly or cream to increase effectiveness. To protect against sexually transmitted diseases and increase efficacy, a condom should be used as well. The diaphragm and cervical cap should be properly fitted and require a doctor's prescription.

Advantages of the diaphragm and cervical cap:

- Safe—no major health concerns.
- Effective (if used with contraceptive jelly or cream).
- Jelly and cream available without a prescription.
- Used only when needed.
- Can be inserted ahead of time.
- Not felt once in place.
- Diaphragm can last for a few years.

Disadvantages and side effects of the diaphragm and cervical cap:

- Skin irritation or allergy to latex or spermicide.
- Recurrent cystitis (infection of the bladder causing frequent and painful urination) with the diaphragm.

- Toxic shock syndrome.
- Requires motivation.
- The method is a little messy.
- Cannot use during vaginal infection.

Note: the diaphragm should be checked by a clinician (fitted) to see if it is still the right size, after a weight change of ten or more pounds, abortion, or childbirth.

SPERMICIDES

Spermicides contain a chemical, usually nonoxynol–9, that kills sperm. They can be obtained in the form of gels, creams, foams, suppositories, or films. Spermicides are usually used together with a barrier method such as a condom or diaphragm to increase protection. You can buy them over the counter without a prescription. As with any other method, always read and follow instructions accurately. Some people are allergic to nonoxynol–9 in spermicides.

Advantages of spermicides:

- Easy to use and cheap.
- Available over the counter.
- Minimal side effects.

Disadvantages of spermicides:

- Should be used together with a barrier method to increase its effectiveness in preventing pregnancy and sexually transmitted diseases.
- Can cause irritation/allergy (rarely).
- Can be messy.
- Requires use every time you have intercourse.

INTRAUTERINE DEVICE (IUD)

A clinician inserts a small device (the IUD) into the uterus. The IUD contains copper or hormones that keep sperm from joining the egg and prevent the fertilized egg from implanting in the uterus. In the United States the IUD is mostly used by women who have completed childbearing, and is rarely used by teenagers. In fact, its use in general has declined dramatically, due to safety concerns relating to the Dalkon Shield. However, the IUD is still used by about 12 percent of women around the world.

Advantages of the IUD:

* Secrecy.
* Minimal effort and demands after insertion.

Disadvantages of the IUD:

* Generally not recommended for adolescents.
* Increased risk of pelvic inflammatory disease in users who develop sexually transmitted diseases.
* Increased risk of infertility as a result of pelvic inflammatory disease.

EMERGENCY CONTRACEPTION (EC)

Contraception used after sex, instead of before, is known as "emergency contraception," or the "morning after pill." It can prevent pregnancy after unprotected vaginal intercourse. This is not the same thing as RU486, the abortion pill. Emergency contraception is no substitute for regular contraception, and is also not as effective as regular contraception. It has, however, been used in cases of rape, cases where a condom has broken, or when contraception has been forgotten. Emergency contraception is a high dose of ordinary birth control pills prescribed by a health-care provider, and must be taken within 72 hours of unprotected sex. Not all birth control pills should be used as emergency contraceptives. Emergency contraception works by preventing ovulation, fertilization, or the implantation of the fertilized egg into the uterus. It decreases a woman's chance of becoming pregnant by about 75 percent. It has no effect once pregnancy has occurred. If you have questions about emergency contraception, your physician should be able to help you. Emergency contraception is available from health-care providers, Planned Parenthood health centers and other women's health and family planning centers. Not all physicians prescribe EC though, so if they can't help, you may call the Emergency Contraceptive hotline at 1-800-584-9911.

WITHDRAWAL METHOD

I mention this because about 4 percent of teenagers rely on this method to prevent pregnancy. The withdrawal method refers to the technique whereby the male withdraws his penis just before his ejaculation, to try to prevent sperm from entering the vagina. Unfortunately this method is not very reliable and it provides no protection against sexually transmitted diseases.

RHYTHM METHOD

This method involves keeping track of a woman's menstrual periods on a calendar, and not having sex around the time of ovulation, when she is most likely to become pregnant. This is not a very effective method of birth control, as it is often difficult to work out exactly when ovulation will occur.

NATURAL FAMILY PLANNING

This is also not a method that is usually recommended for teenagers. Natural family planning involves keeping a chart of a woman's daily body temperature and the type of mucus she secretes, in order to determine when she is ovulating.

STERILIZATION METHODS

These include tubal ligation and vasectomy. Because many people change their minds about wanting to have children, sterilization is not usually recommended for people under the age of 30 who have not had children.

TUBAL LIGATION

This surgical procedure is intended to permanently block a woman's tubes, where the sperm joins the egg.

VASECTOMY

This is an operation which is intended to permanently block a man's tubes (the vas deferens) through which the sperm travels, so that pregnancy can't occur. This does not prevent sperm from being produced.

Once-a-Month Contraception

The FDA has also approved the first once-a-month contraceptive, marketed as Lunelle, which is a combination of progestin and estrogen. Compared with Depo-Provera, which has progestin only, and is given every three months, Lunelle allows a woman to have a more regular menstrual cycle, and return to fertility more rapidly (Guttmacher Report, Dec., 2000).

Costs of Contraception

This information was obtained in part from the Planned Parenthood website.

Note: about a third of insurance providers cover contraceptive costs at this time. Hopefully, more will do so in the future.

• Oral contraceptives: about $360 per year with no prescription coverage. Costs $15–30 per pack of pills at drugstores and usually less at clinics, and you have to factor in the cost of an examination.
• Diaphragm: Out-of-pocket expense for a diaphragm is about $200 per year with no prescription plan.
• Condoms and spermicide: 25–50¢ per condom—depends on need. Not covered by any insurance plan at this time.
• Injectable Depo-Provera: $180 per year with no prescription plan.
• Norplant: around $450 with no prescription plan.

Although contraception costs some money, the costs of an unwanted pregnancy and associated problems are much greater!

"Near-Misses"

I interviewed a large number of young people, both men and women, while working on this book, and on several occasions I came upon the term "near-miss," usually in my interviews with men. I was talking to Mike, who is now 25 years old, and he told me that he had never "got a girl pregnant." He went on to say: "I've had a few near-misses though." He explained to me that a "near-miss" was a close call, when the girl thought she might be pregnant, and then found out she wasn't.

Why do some people require a dramatic event in order to change their ways for the better? For example, why do some people wait until they have a heart attack, before they stop smoking or take their medicine for high cholesterol? As a doctor I've seen this happen over and over again. Until it hits really close to home, one doesn't believe it could happen to them. By the way some people don't ever learn. I'll never forget visiting a man who had just recovered from a heart attack. He was sitting in his hospital bed smoking!

In the case of teenage pregnancy, Mike admitted to having more than one "near-miss." Shouldn't one scare a person enough to make sure that they are either abstinent or using contraception regularly? Unfortunately for many, it takes a real pregnancy before it hits home. Don't let that happen to you.

Male Reproductive Health Care

A sexual relationship and its consequences should really be the responsibility of both partners, but unfortunately reproductive health care and support services for men are lacking. Teenage males in the United States do not routinely receive reproductive health services such as counseling by a medical professional and testing for sexually transmitted diseases. If men came to a clinic specifically for those tests, they would be done, but routinely they don't.

Because of the high rate of unwanted pregnancies and sexually transmitted diseases in the U.S., I hope that it will become more routine for doctors to counsel on sexual health and prevention to all teenagers, both male and female.

Oral Sex

There are some reports that oral sex is becoming more common among teenagers, but this has not been substantiated. It makes sense, that because teenagers are aware that sex can cause unwanted pregnancies and sexually transmitted diseases, some teenagers will consider engaging in sexual activity which they believe puts them at less risk.

However, teenagers may not have been given all the facts. Oral sex may not put them at risk of pregnancy, but sexually transmitted diseases can be caused by sexual activity other than intercourse. So now defining sex starts to become important. It's important for you as a teenager to talk to your doctor about how to protect yourself if you are involved in any kind of sexual activity.

In general, helping young people prevent an unintended pregnancy should be an important goal to all of us, including teenagers themselves. It will not only prevent the often negative effects of teenage childbearing on young women and their children, but will decrease the high incidence of abortions and the high costs to society. Numerous efforts are being undertaken, with increasing education about abstinence and contraception and the value of delaying sexual activity. Community partnerships in a number of states have developed comprehensive youth programs to prevent teenage pregnancies and related problems. When we look at the decline in the rates of teenage pregnancy and abortions between 1991 and 1996, it seems as if these efforts are paying off.

STOP!

Before you decide to have a sexual relationship, remember:

- Sex is not the same thing as love and intimacy.
- Sex cannot buy love or make someone love you.
- Sex will not guarantee that your partner will stay with you forever.
- You decide when you are ready for a sexual relationship.

Sexually transmitted diseases

"Against diseases here the strongest fence
Is the defensive virtue, Abstinence"
—Robert Herrick (1591–1674)

Sexually transmitted diseases, previously known as venereal diseases, are among the most common infectious diseases in the U.S. today. They are infections spread by sexual contact, including vaginal, anal, and oral sex. Three million teenagers are infected with a sexually transmitted disease every year.

Here are the important facts about most sexually transmitted diseases:

1. Sexually transmitted diseases affect men and women of all backgrounds. They are most prevalent among teenagers and young adults. The rate of gonorrhea, for example, is highest among females aged 15 to 19 years (CDC-MMWR, 1998). Some reasons for this higher risk are that teenagers are biologically more susceptible to certain infections, they may have unprotected intercourse, and they may not be able to obtain health care early.

2. The incidence of sexually transmitted diseases is rising. Reasons for this include people becoming sexually active at a younger age, yet marrying later, and divorce becoming more common. As a result of these, people are more likely to have multiple sex partners during their lives, and this increases their risk of acquiring an STD.

3. Sexually transmitted diseases often remain undiagnosed because symptoms may not be recognized as such or because STDs may produce no symptoms, especially in women. The problem is that even if an infected

person has no symptoms, they can still pass the disease on to a sex partner. For this reason it is very important for all sexually active people to have routine screenings for sexually transmitted diseases.

4. Complications of STDs can be serious, especially for women, in whom the diagnosis is sometimes made late.

• Some STDs can spread, causing pelvic inflammatory disease (PID), which can lead to infertility and ectopic (tubal) pregnancy, which can be fatal.

• Human papillomavirus is associated with cancer of the cervix.

• STDs can be passed from a mother to her baby before or during birth, or through breastfeeding.

5. When diagnosed early, many sexually transmitted diseases can be treated effectively.

I'm writing about sexually transmitted diseases in this book because if you are, or have ever been, sexually active, you have put yourself at risk of having a sexually transmitted disease. If teenagers have all the knowledge and facts, they may make the correct decisions about their health.

In this chapter I try to give information about sexually transmitted diseases, so you can decide how best to protect yourself. If you have been exposed, go for diagnosis and treatment early.

There are many important things to know:

• You should learn how to decrease your risk for sexually transmitted diseases (STDs).

• You should understand the importance of being tested, because not all sexually transmitted diseases cause obvious symptoms.

• You should know how and where to get treatment.

• You should be aware that if you do have a sexually transmitted disease, your sexual partner should be counseled and treated too. This will prevent reinfection or the spread of infection.

More facts and statistics:

• One quarter of all sexually active teenagers are infected with a sexually transmitted disease before they complete high school.

• Two-thirds of twelfth graders have had sexual intercourse.

• Fifty percent of teenagers say they used no birth control the first time they had sex, and only a third of all sexually active teenagers routinely use contraception.

The Most Common Sexually Transmitted Diseases

HIV

Acquired immunodeficiency syndrome (AIDS) was first reported in the U.S. in 1981. It is caused by the HIV virus, which destroys the body's ability to fight off infection. About 900,000 people in the U.S. are currently infected with HIV. Transmission of the virus occurs primarily during sexual activity and through sharing needles used to inject intravenous drugs. Infection with HIV can produce a spectrum of disease ranging from no symptoms at all to having AIDS. The time between being infected with the virus and development of AIDS ranges from a few months to many years. AIDS eventually develops in almost all HIV-infected people, but early diagnosis is still essential because there are now treatments available to slow the disease process. Treatment is also available to prevent complicating infections, and early diagnosis prevents the spread of the disease.

It is reassuring to know that you don't get AIDS from casual contact; for example, from touching objects or people, or being around an infected person, or shaking hands with them, or using the same bathroom as them.

AIDS is spread by:

• Sexual intercourse with an infected person. people of either sex can pass the disease to the other party.

• Intravenous needles: The virus can be passed through sharing needles used to inject illegal drugs.

• Blood transfusions: It is now very rare to get AIDS from a blood transfusion, as all blood is screened for the HIV virus. It is also important to know that you can't get AIDS from donating blood.

• Pregnant woman to infant: An infected pregnant woman can pass the AIDS virus into her unborn baby's blood stream.

For more information, the AIDS Hotline toll-free number is 1-800-342-AIDS.

GENITAL HERPES SIMPLEX VIRUS (HSV) INFECTION

Genital herpes is caused by herpes simplex types 1 and 2. Type 2 more commonly causes genital lesions, while type 1 causes sores around the mouth. Genital herpes is a recurrent viral infection. Once you get the virus, it remains in your body always, resurfacing at times to cause new outbreaks. Symptoms include sore blisters, which form ulcers. The blisters may be preceded by a tingling or burning sensation. Fever may also develop with the first episode. Some cases of first-episode infections are severe enough to require hospitalization. Many people have no symptoms, but may still spread the virus to others.

To date there is no cure, but treatment with medication can help control symptoms. Severe or frequent recurrent genital herpes is treated with one of several antiviral drugs that are available by prescription. Condoms help prevent spread of infection.

A mother infected with the herpes virus can pass it on to her baby in the birth process. Herpes simplex infection acquired in the newborn period can be extremely serious. Infants can become very ill if not treated promptly, and are also much more likely to be born prematurely. Some of the ways newborns can present with herpes are the following:

• Disease involving multiple organs, including the liver and the lungs.
• Central nervous system disease.
• Disease of the skin, eyes and mouth. In about 40 percent of cases, the skin, eyes, and mouth are affected.
• Without skin lesions the diagnosis of herpes simplex infection in a newborn can be very difficult, so it is important to notify your doctor if you have any known history of herpes.
• Babies with fever, irritability and seizures should also be checked for herpes.

The risk of an infected mother passing the herpes simplex virus to her baby is high if she acquires the infection near the time of delivery (30–50 percent) and low in women who acquire the infection early in pregnancy or have recurrent herpes. It's important to avoid unprotected genital and oral sexual contact during pregnancy, especially late pregnancy, unless you are in a stable relationship with a partner who you know is uninfected.

CHLAMYDIA

Chlamydia is a bacterial infection which affects between four and eight million people in the United States each year. It is the most commonly reported sexually transmitted infection in the U.S. Its prevalence in pregnant women in general varies between 6 and 12 percent, but in pregnant teenagers, the prevalence can be as high as 37 percent.

Symptoms in women include abnormal vaginal discharge, irregular bleeding, lower abdominal pain, or painful or frequent urination. Chlamydia is sometimes called the "silent epidemic," because in women it is also not unusual to have no symptoms at all. These women still develop complications, so if you are sexually active, it is important to be screened for chlamydia. Men may develop burning on urination, penile discharge, or discomfort in the abdomen or testicles during intercourse.

Chlamydia is treatable with antibiotics. If untreated, it can cause pelvic inflammatory disease (PID), which can lead to sterility, ectopic pregnancy, or chronic pelvic pain. If you are infected with chlamydia during pregnancy, treatment can also prevent the spread of the infection to your baby during birth. Chlamydia also causes complications in men.

Gonorrhea

In the United States about 600,000 new infections of gonorrhea occur each year. Women may complain of pain, abnormal vaginal discharge, or bleeding. In teenage girls, gonorrheal infection is most often asymptomatic. Men may have burning on urination, penile discharge, or pain. Gonorrhea may also infect the rectum, throat and eyes.

Gonorrhea is treatable with antibiotics. If untreated, even asymptomatic infection can cause serious complications, which in women include pelvic inflammatory disease, infertility, and ectopic pregnancy. Because infections in women are often asymptomatic, it is important to be screened for this infection.

Genital Warts

Genital warts are caused by human papillomavirus (HPV), which is a virus similar to the one causing warts on the skin. Genital warts generally occur as small painless lesions in the genital area. Most infections are unrecognized. There are many strains of HPV (more than 20 types can affect the genital tract). Some strains have been strongly associated with cervical dysplasia and cervical cancer. Because HPV is contagious, often asymptomatic, and may increase one's risk for developing cervical cancer, it's important to be checked regularly and have a pap smear every year. Genital warts are treated by various methods, including with a topical drug (applied to the skin), by freezing, or by surgery.

SYPHILIS

Syphilis is a bacterial infection which progresses over time and can cause permanent damage if untreated. The infection can be divided into three stages. The first stage appears as one or more painless sores or ulcers of the skin and mucous membranes, most often in the genital area. Lymph nodes in the area become swollen. The secondary stage usually manifests with a skin rash, about one to two months later. The third stage can affect other systems including the heart and the nervous system. Syphilis is easily diagnosed with a blood test and is treatable with antibiotics if they are given early in the disease. All pregnant women should be tested for syphilis, as it can cause serious problems in newborns.

HEPATITIS B

Hepatitis B is a viral infection, which in the decade preceding 1998, infected about 240,000 people in the U.S. each year. Hopefully with increased use of the hepatitis B vaccine, the incidence will decrease dramatically. Hepatitis B virus is transmitted through blood or body fluids, such as semen, cervical secretions, saliva, and wound exudate. About 30 to 60 percent of cases are sexually transmitted. The virus can also be transmitted from an infected mother to her baby. Transmission through blood products is now rare in the U.S., because of routine screening of blood for infection. Hepatitis B virus causes a wide spectrum of symptoms and illness, ranging from minimal or no symptoms to fatal hepatitis. There is no cure for acute hepatitis B at this time, although medications are used to control it.

The good news is that there is a very effective vaccine which can prevent infection. The series consists of three shots and has a good safety record in children. To eventually eliminate transmission of hepatitis B virus, universal immunization is necessary. Hepatitis B vaccine is recommended for all infants as part of their routine immunization series, and all children who have not received the vaccine previously should be immunized by or before 12 years of age.

TRICHOMONIASIS

This infection affects about three million people per year. It is primarily transmitted sexually and often coexists with other sexually transmitted diseases such as gonorrhea. Women may develop vaginal discharge or itching, painful intercourse, or frequent urination. Men may have no symptoms, frequent urination, or penile discharge. Infection in men is often mild and self-limited. Trichomoniasis is treatable with medication.

BACTERIAL VAGINOSIS

Bacterial vaginosis has also been known as "Gardnerella" or "Moraxella." This bacterial infection occurs especially in sexually active adolescent and young adult women. The usual symptoms include a white vaginal discharge with a fishy odor, but the infection may be asymptomatic.

SCABIES

These are mites that spread from person to person through prolonged, close contact, including but not only sexual contact. Symptoms include intense itching of the skin, especially at night. Topical treatments are available to treat scabies.

CHANCROID

Chancroid is an infection transmitted exclusively through sexual contact. It causes ulceration of the genital area. Men usually have a single ulcer, while women have many lesions. The ulcer that develops in chancroid, unlike syphilis, is painful and tender. Women may also present with less obvious symptoms such as vaginal discharge or burning on urination; they may even be asymptomatic.

OTHER STDS

Several other less common diseases are transmitted through sexual contact, including lymphogranuloma venereum, and granuloma inguinale.

Lymphogranuloma venereum: This is one of the clinical presentations of chlamydia. Women often have no symptoms. The infection can be transmitted during the active stage which may last from weeks to many years.

Granulome inguinale: This disease is caused by a bacterium Calymmatobacterium granulomatis. This no longer occurs in the United States and most developed countries, but we do see this in people coming in from other parts of the world, including New Guinea, India and Africa.

Pelvic inflammatory disease is a spectrum of inflammatory disorders of the female upper genital tract, most commonly seen among teenagers and young adults. The most common infections causing this are gonorrhea and chlamydia. It typically causes dull, continuous abdominal or pelvic pain, that may be anything from mild to severe. Other symptoms include fever, vomiting, abnormal vaginal discharge, or irregular bleeding. Pelvic inflammatory disease may also occur without symptoms at all, and so many episodes go unrecognized. This becomes a major problem, as the complications, if untreated, are very serious. These include abscess, ectopic pregnancy, infertility, and chronic pain.

Sexual Partners and STDs

It is very important to know the sexual history of a potential sex partner. To be on the safe side, it is best that you both get tested for sexually transmitted diseases, including HIV, before you begin a sexual relationship. Know that tests may not detect HIV if less than six months has passed since the time of infection.

SEXUAL ASSAULT AND STDS

Infections seen most commonly in women and young girls who have been sexually assaulted are trichomoniasis, bacterial vaginosis, chlamydia, and gonorrhea. HIV is also a great concern. I mention sexual assault, because it does happen, and many times even goes unreported. Seek help immediately! Some doctors recommend routine preventive therapy after an assault.

Sexually Transmitted Diseases in Pregnancy

Women who are pregnant can become infected with the same STDs as women who are not pregnant. Pregnancy provides no protection from

STDs for either women or their babies. Instead, STDs can have very serious effects on a pregnant woman and the fetus.

For the mother, many complications are similar to those occurring in women who are not pregnant. STDs are associated with liver problems and some cancers, among other problems. Pregnant women may go into labor early and give birth to small babies, or may develop uterine infection after delivery.

STDs can be transmitted from a pregnant woman to her baby, before, during or after birth. The effects on a baby can be very serious and include congenital abnormalities, hepatitis, pneumonia, and even stillbirth.

For the above reasons, if you are pregnant, you should be screened for sexually transmitted diseases, particularly gonorrhea, chlamydia, hepatitis B, HIV and syphilis (CDC STD Treatment Guidelines, 1997).

Prevention of STDs

Nothing is as effective as abstinence when it comes to preventing pregnancy or sexually transmitted diseases. Short of that, the best way to prevent a sexually transmitted disease, including AIDS, is not to have sex with an infected partner.

If you do decide to have sexual intercourse:

1. Have a monogamous sexual relationship with a partner who is not infected. You and your partner should be tested for STDs, including HIV, before beginning the sexual relationship.

2. Using a condom correctly every time you have sex can also help to decrease the risk of STDs. Here are some tips on correct use:
   • Use a new condom each time you have sex.
   • Handle the condom carefully to avoid damage to it.
   • The condom should be put on an erect penis and before any genital contact.
   • No air should be trapped in the tip of the condom.
   • Only water-based lubricants such as K-Y jelly should be used with latex condoms. Oil-based lubricants can weaken latex.

3. Hepatitis B can be sexually transmitted, so check with your doctor about getting the hepatitis B vaccine if you are unvaccinated.

4. Delay having sexual relationships as long as possible.

If you are diagnosed with a sexually transmitted disease:

1. Get treated as soon as possible. It's important to know that with very few exceptions, all teenagers in the United States can give consent to the confidential diagnosis and treatment of STDs. You do not need the consent of your parents in order to get treated. (See "Minors and the right to consent to health care" below.)

2. Notify all recent sexual contacts and urge them to get checked.

3. Complete the full course of medication as per the doctor's instructions. Follow up as necessary.

4. Avoid sexual activity while being treated.

5. If you are breastfeeding, discuss with your doctor whether the infection is transmitted through breast milk and whether formula should be substituted.

Minors and the Right to Consent to Health Care

It has been well established, in federal and state policy, that many minors have the capacity and even the right to make important decisions about their health care. Many states specifically authorize minors to consent to contraceptive services, testing and treatment for sexually transmitted diseases including HIV, and treatment for drug and alcohol abuse, amongst other things. In the case of abortion, lawmakers have and will continue to try to impose various restrictions on this right. These restrictions may be in the form of parental consent or notification requirements.

Establishing rules for the consent of minors is a very difficult and controversial issue that faces lawmakers. On the one hand, it seems reasonable that parents should have the right and the responsibility to make health-care decisions for their minor child. On the other hand, in certain situations, it may be more important for a young person to have access to confidential medical services.

Some teenagers who are sexually active, pregnant, or infected with a sexually transmitted disease, and those who abuse drugs or alcohol, may not seek care if they must involve their parents. Finding the right balance between the rights of minors and their parents' rights, will continue to be a topic for debate.

If you need more information about STDs, contact your private doctor, local health department, or an STD or family planning clinic.

Conclusion

Despite the recent decline in teen pregnancy and birth rates, teenage pregnancy still remains a significant problem in the U.S. Too many American girls are negatively affected by an early pregnancy. It strongly impacts not only their lives, but their families and their communities.

Although sexual activity among teenagers and teenage pregnancy are not unique to this era, the following changes have occurred in the last few decades.

- The average age of menarche (onset of menstruation) has decreased.
- Teenagers are having sex at an earlier age.
- People are marrying later.

Because of these factors, more young people are sexually experienced. In addition, more are sexually active before marriage and have more than one partner before marriage. We are therefore seeing higher rates of unwanted pregnancies, single parenthood, and sexually transmitted diseases.

Media portrayals of sex are not helping matters. Television and movies often depict beautiful unmarried people having sex. They rarely discuss contraception or the consequences such as pregnancy and sexually transmitted diseases.

As a teenager, what can you do?

1. You have a long exciting road ahead of you, with potential for a great future. Know that you have the ability to make decisions now that will shape your future.

2. Remember that having a sexual relationship does not ensure love, and having a baby with someone does not ensure that a relationship will

stay intact. Hold off on sexual relationships until you are in a committed, loving relationship to avoid paying a high emotional price later.

3. Be educated about the prevention of pregnancy and sexually transmitted diseases, including AIDS. Knowledge gives you the power to make good decisions.

4. Communicate with your parents more openly if possible. Just as it may be difficult for teenagers to discuss sex and contraception with their parents, for many parents it is difficult to broach this topic with their children. Parents often hope that it will be covered adequately at school. However, it is important that you all try. Talk about the facts, and also ask your parents about their values and moral beliefs.

5. Get involved in community issues and in promoting responsible media. Television, for example, should include more realistic storylines about sex and its consequences.

My hope is that the teenagers of today and tomorrow will take control of their lives in a positive way, and so further reduce the incidence of unwanted pregnancies, and also sexually transmitted diseases.

Being a pregnant teenager need not be a hopeless situation. You are young and you still have many choices to make. You may choose to continue your schooling or go to college. You may choose to remain single or to marry. You can still find your life to be rewarding and challenging in many ways. Although your pregnancy was unplanned, you can learn and mature from your situation. You are in a position to make decisions for yourself, and you still have the opportunity to accomplish great things in life. You can help break the cycle of poverty and diminished education that is all too common amongst teenage mothers. You can set higher goals. I hope this book will help you do so.

Appendix A:
Pregnancy Action Plan

You suspect that you are pregnant.

Confirm pregnancy with a pregnancy test:

If the test is negative and you have confirmed this:
Review your situation. Taking into account unwanted pregnancies and sexually transmitted disease, is it really your choice to be sexually active at this time? If not, delaying further sex until you are ready will decrease your risks for both problems. If you decide to be sexually active, make sure your contraceptive method is reliable and that you are using it correctly.

If your pregnancy test is positive:
1. Talk to someone you trust: your parents, partner, other family member, counselor, member of the clergy, or another trusted adult.
2. Schedule an appointment with a doctor or health-care provider as soon as possible, or visit your local Planned Parenthood Center for help.
3. Get complete information about all your pregnancy options: parenting, adoption, and abortion.
4. Speak to a counselor if necessary.
5. Establish legal paternity.
6. Choose one of your three options.

None of these options is easy, so before making your decision, make sure you have all the facts, have reviewed all the possibilities, and feel comfortable about your decision. There is always someone who can help you and guide you. You must never feel alone. It is not a sign of weakness to ask for help or see a counselor. It's often a very wise decision.

If you choose **PARENTING***:*

1. Have a checkup with an obstetrician-gynecologist or other health-care provider as soon as possible.

2. Take care of yourself and your unborn baby. Do not smoke, drink alcohol, or take illegal drugs. Check with your doctor about any other medications you might be taking, including prescription or over-the-counter medications.

3. Go for regular checkups to keep yourself healthy during your pregnancy and to increase the chances of having a healthy baby.

4. Decide whether you will parent with or without a partner, and if you will marry or not.

5. Decide whether you will parent with the help of your parents or another family member.

6. Plan your education: Consider whether you will continue with your schooling or career at this time, or put it on hold until later.

7. Look at your finances. Moving in with your parents on a short-term basis can help save costs.

8. Take a parenting class.

9. Consider joining a support group.

10. Set goals for your future.

If you choose **ADOPTION***:*

1. Speak to your partner, your parents, another family member, or other trusted adult.

2. Have a checkup with an obstetrician-gynecologist or another health-care provider as soon as possible.

3. Do not smoke, drink alcohol, or take illegal drugs. Check with your doctor about any other medication you may be taking.

4. Go for regular checkups to keep yourself healthy during your pregnancy, and to increase your chances of giving birth to a healthy baby.

5. Read about adoption.

6. Decide on an agency versus an independent adoption. If you choose an independent adoption, find a reputable adoption attorney who has your interests at heart.

7. Schedule an appointment with the agency or the adoption attorney.

8. Learn about the adoption laws in your state, including how to involve the birthfather legally.

9. Take advantage of pre- and post-adoption counseling.

10. Decide about closed versus open adoption. Your counselor will give you more information about these options.

11. Join a birthparents support group.

12. Set goals for your future.

If you choose **ABORTION***:*

The decision to abort needs to be made relatively early in your pregnancy, as the earlier an abortion is done, the safer the procedure is, and after a certain time in your pregnancy, an abortion can no longer be performed.

1. Speak to your parents and to your partner to the extent that you are able. Check on the abortion laws regarding parental notification and consent in your state.

2. Schedule an appointment with your doctor, or with a healthcare provider or clinic that provides abortion services. A good place to go for help might be your local Planned Parenthood affiliate. Call 1-800-230-PLAN.

3. Enlist the support of your family and the baby's father if possible.

4. Take advantage of counseling.

5. Schedule and keep a follow-up appointment with your healthcare provider, so they can make sure you are well, to answer any questions you might have, and to discuss post-abortion contraception with you if you plan to continue to be sexually active.

Appendix B: Resources

This is really a book about getting the help you need, so I hope you make use of some of the resources I have included. There are resources for pregnant women, their partners, families, and teachers. There are also resources for single dads. You can also check their websites for more information, free publications, and support groups which may be available to you in your area. I have included more detailed information on some of the groups and agencies where available.

General Health and Social Services Information

Alan Guttmacher Institute
Tel: 202-296-4012
http://www.agi-usa.org
The Alan Guttmacher Institute provides reliable nonpartisan information on sexual activity, contraception, abortion, and childbearing. It provides most of its information through its journals, its public policy reviews, and its website.

American Academy of Pediatrics
www.aap.org

Center for Disease Control
Atlanta, Georgia
Tel: 1-888-232-3278

National STD hotline: 1-800-227-8922
www.cdc.gov/nchs

American College of Obstetricians and Gynecologists
409 12th Street, SW
P.O. Box 96920
Washington, D.C. 20090–6920
Tel: 202-638-5577
www.acog.com

Rape Abuse and Incest National Network (RAINN) Hotline
Tel: 800-656-HOPE

American Social Health Association
P.O. Box 13827
Research Triangle Park, NC 27709
Tel: 919-361-8400
www.ashastd.org

New York Online Access to Health (NOAH)
www.noah-health.org
   This is a bilingual (English and Spanish) health information site.

Sexuality Information and Education Council of the United States (SIECUS)
130 West 42nd Street, Suite 350
New York, NY 10036–7802
Tel: 212-819-9770
www.siecus.org

National Council on Family Relations
3989 Central Ave., NE, Suite 550
Minneapolis, MN 55421
Tel: 888-781-9331
www.ncfr.com

Center for Reproductive Law and Policy
120 Wall Street
18th Floor
New York, NY 10005
Tel: 917-637-3600

Pregnancy Prevention

The National Campaign to Prevent Teen Pregnancy
1776 Mass. Ave., NW, Suite 200
Washington, D.C. 20036
Tel: 202-478-8500
www.teenpregnancy.org

Founded in 1996, the National Campaign to Prevent Teen Pregnancy is a nonprofit, nonpartisan initiative, supported entirely by private donations. Its mission is to prevent teenage pregnancy by supporting values and stimulating actions that are consistent with a pregnancy-free adolescence.

Planned Parenthood Federation of America
810 Seventh Ave., New York, N.Y., 10019
Tel: 800-230-PLAN

Planned Parenthood is the largest voluntary family planning organization. They uphold the principle that every individual has a fundamental right to decide when or whether to have a child, and that every child should be wanted and loved. Planned Parenthood provides reproductive and complementary health-care services through its network of affiliates nationwide.

D.C. Community Prevention Partnership
1612 K Street, NW, Suite 1100
Washington, D.C. 20006
Tel: 202-898-4700

Emergency Contraception Hotline
Tel: 800-584-9911

**National Organization on Adolescent Pregnancy, Parenting
and Prevention**
1319 F Street, NW, Suite 400
Washington, D.C. 20004
Tel: 202-783-5770

Abortion

National Abortion Federation
1436 U Street, NW, Suite 103
Washington, D.C. 20009
Hotline: 800-772-9100
   The National Abortion Federation Hotline provides callers with factual information about abortions in both English and Spanish.

National Abortion and Reproductive Rights Action League (NARAL)
1156 15th Street, NW
7th Floor
Washington, D.C. 20005
Tel: 202-973-3000
www. naral.org

Adoption

Adoptions Together, Inc. (private adoption agency)
10230 New Hampshire Ave., Suite 200
Silver Spring, MD 20903
Tel: 301-439-2900
Tel: 800-439-0233

Resolve
Tel: 617-623-0744
   National Helpline offering advice and support with infertility issues and adoption.

National Adoption Information Clearinghouse
330 C Street, SW
Washington, D.C. 20447
Tel: 703-352-3488
Tel: 888-251-0075
www.calib.com/naic

NAIC is a comprehensive resource on all aspects of adoption. It is a service of the Children's Bureau, Administration on Children, Youth and Families, Administration for Children and Families, Dept. of Health and Human Services.

National Council for Adoption
1930 Seventeenth Street, NW
Washington, D.C. 20009
Tel: 202-328-1200

American Academy of Adoption Attorneys
P.O. Box 33053
Washington D.C. 20033–0053
Tel: 202-832-2222

American Adoption Congress
P.O. Box 42730
Washington, D.C. 20015
Tel: 202-483-3399
www.americanadoptioncongress.org

Concerned United Birthparents
2000 Walker Street
Des Moines, IA 50317
Tel: 800-822-2777

Parenting

Active Parenting Publishers
810 Franklin Court, Suite B
Marietta, GA 30067
Tel: 800-825-0060
www.activeparenting.com

References

Books

Adamec, Christine. *The Adoption Option: Complete Handbook 2000–2001*. Roseville, CA: Prima, 1999.

American Academy of Child and Adolescent Psychiatry. *Your Adolescent*. New York, NY: HarperResource, 1999

Anderson, Joan. *The Single Mother's Book: A Practical Guide to Managing Your Children, Career, Home, Finances, and Everything Else*. Atlanta, GA: Peachtree, 1990.

Arthur, Shirley. *Surviving Teen Pregnancy*. Revised. Buena Park, CA: Morning Glory, 1996.

Boston Women's Health Book Collective. *Our Bodies Ourselves for the New Century: A Book by and for Women*. New York, NY: Simon and Schuster, 1998.

Buckingham, Robert W., and Mary Derby. *I'm Pregnant, Now What Do I Do?* Amherst, NY: Prometheus Books, 1997.

Coles, Robert. *The Youngest Parents*. New York, NY: W.W. Norton, 1997.

Covey, Stephen R. *The 7 Habits of Highly Effective Families*. New York, NY: Golden, 1997.

DelleVecchio, Andrea. *The Unofficial Guide to Adopting a Child*. Foster City, CA: IDG Books Worldwide, 2000.

Engber, Andrea, and Leah Klungness. *The Complete Single Mother: Reassuring Answers to Your Most Challenging Concerns*. Holbrook, MA: Adams, 1995, 2000.

Foge, Leslie, and Gail Mosconi. *The Third Choice: A Woman's Guide to Placing a Child for Adoption*. Berkeley, CA: Creative Arts, 1999.

Gilman, Lois. *The Adoption Resource Book*. 4th Edition. New York, NY: HarperPerennial, 1998.

Gritter, James L. *The Spirit of Open Adoption*. Washington, D.C.: Child Welfare League of America, 1997.

Lerman, Evelyn. *Teen Moms: The Pain and the Promise*. Buena Park, CA: Morning Glory, 1997.

Lieberman, E. James, and Karen Lieberman Troccoli. *Like It Is: A Teen Sex Guide*. Jefferson, NC: McFarland, 1998.

Lindsay, Jeanne Warren. *Pregnant? Adoption Is an Option*. Buena Park, CA: Morning Glory, 1997.

Luker, Kristin. *Dubious Conceptions: The Politics of Teenage Pregnancy*. Cambridge, MA.: Harvard University Press, 1996

Salk, Lee. *Familyhood: Nurturing the Values That Matter*. New York, NY: Simon and Schuster, 1992.

Sherman, Aliza. *Everything You Need to Know About Placing Your Baby for Adoption*. New York, NY: The Rosen Publishing Group, 1996.

Thompson, Stephen P., editor. *Teenage Pregnancy Opposing Viewpoints*. San Diego, CA: David L. Bender, Greenhaven, 1997.

Torre-Bueno, Ava. *Peace After Abortion*. San Diego, CA: Pimpernel, 1997.

Articles

ACOG News Release. Pharmacists Limit Women's Access to Emergency Contraception. May 1999

Alan Guttmacher Institute. Facts in Brief. Contraceptive Use. 1998.

The Alan Guttmacher Institute—Occasional report. Darroch JE, Singh S. Why Is Teenage Pregnancy Declining? The Roles of Abstinence, Sexual Activity and Contraceptive Use. 1999

American Academy of Pediatrics: Red Book 2000. Report of the Committee on Infectious Diseases. 25th edition.

American Academy of Pediatrics-Committee on Adolescence. Adolescent Pregnancy-Current Trends and Issues:1998. *Pediatrics*. Feb. 1999; 103(2) 516–20

American Academy of Pediatrics—Committee on Adolescence. Contraception and Adolescents. *Pediatrics*. Nov. 1999; 104(5): 1161–66

American Academy of Pediatrics—Committee on Adolescence. Counseling the Adolescent about Pregnancy Options. *Pediatrics*. May 1998; 101(5) 938–40

CDC MMWR. 1998 Guidelines for Treatment of Sexually Transmitted Diseases. Jan. 1998; 47(RR-1)

Darroch, J.E., Landry, D.J., Singh S. Changing Emphases in Sexuality Education in U.S. Public Secondary Schools, 1988–1999. *Family Planning Perspectives*. Sept/Oct 2000; 32(5)

Family Planning Perspectives. Reproductive Health Services Typically Are Not Part of Male Teenagers' Routine Medical Care. Nov/Dec 2000; 32(6)

Family Planning Perspectives. U.S. Births Rise for First Time in Eight Years. Births to Teenagers Still Falling. Sept/Oct 2000; 32(5)

Ford, C.A., Bearman P.S., Moody M. Foregone Health Care Among Adolescents. *JAMA*. Dec. 1999; 282(23) 2227–34

Guttmacher Report. Dec. 2000

Guttmacher Report on Public Policy. June 2000; 3(3)

Hacker, R.A., Amare, Y., Strunk, N., Horst, L. Listening to Youth. Teen Perspectives on Pregnancy Prevention. *J. Adolescent Health*. April 2000; 26(4) 279–88

Hall, R.T. Prevention of Premature Birth: Do Pediatricians Have a Role? *Pediatrics*. May 2000; 105(5) 1137–40

Hall, R.T., Carroll, R.E. Infant Feeding. *Pediatrics in Review*. June 2000; 21(6) 191–200

Heneghan, A.M., Silver, E.J., Bauman, L.J., Westbrook, L.E., Stein, R.E.K. Depressive Symptoms in Inner-City Mothers of Young Children: Who Is at Risk? *Pediatrics*. Dec. 1998; 102(6) 1394–1400

Jaskiewicz, J.A., McAnarney, E.R. Pregnancy During Adolescence. *Pediatrics in Review*. Jan. 1994; 15: 32–38

Kaiser Daily HIV/AIDS Report. Teens Sexual Decisions Based Mainly on School Performance, Friends. Dec 2000

Kaufmann, R.B., et al. The Decline in U.S. Teen Pregnancy Rates, 1990–1995. *Pediatrics*. Nov. 1998; 102(5) 1141–47

Kinsman, S.B., Romer, D., Furstenberg, F.F., Schwartz, D.F. Early Sexual Initiation: The Role of Peer Norms. *Pediatrics*. Nov. 1998; 102(5) 1185–92

Kirby, D. No Easy Answers. Research Findings on Programs to Reduce Teen Pregnancy. The National Campaign to Prevent Teen Pregnancy. March 1997.

Lappa, S., Moscicki, A.B. The Pediatrician and the Sexually Active Adolescent. *Pediatric Clinics of North America*. Dec. 1997; 44(6)

Lieberman, E.J., Whipple, K. Adoption and Mental Health. *Friend of the Court*. Spring 1997; Vol.5

Lucassen, P.L.B.J., Assendelft, W.J.J., Gubbels, J.W., van Eijk, J.Th.M., Douwes, A.C. Infantile Colic: Crying Time Reduction with a Whey Hydrolysate: A Double-Blind, Randomized, Placebo-Controlled Trial. *Pediatrics*. Dec. 2000; 106(6) 1349–54

McDermott, M.T. Agency Versus Independent Adoption: The Case for Independent Adoption. The Future of Children. *Adoption*. Published by the David and Lucile Packard Foundation. Spring 1993; 3(1)

McDermott, M.T. Avoiding Contested Adoptions. Resolve of the Washington Metropolitan Area, Inc. Nov/Dec 1993

McDermott, M.T. Is Directed Agency Placement the Right Choice? *Face Facts*. May/June 1995

McDermott, M.T. Uniform Adoption Law Offers Hope. Resolve of the Washington Metropolitan Area, Inc. March/April 1996

Miller, F.C. Impact of Adolescent Pregnancy as We Approach the New Millennium. *J. Pediatr. Adolesc. Gynecol*. Feb 2000; 13(1) 5–8

Moore, K.A., Driscoll, A.K., Lindberg, L.D. A Statistical Portrait of Adolescent Sex,

Contraception, and Childbearing. The National Campaign to Prevent Teen Pregnancy. March 1998

The National Campaign to Prevent Teen Pregnancy. Campaign Update. Summer 1999 Adoption Quarterly. Innovations in Community and Clinical Practice, Theory and Research. Published by Haworth Press, Inc. 2000; 3(4)

The National Campaign to Prevent Teen Pregnancy. Whatever Happened to Childhood? The Problem of Teen Pregnancy in the United States. May 1997

Newacheck, P.W., et al. Adolescent Health: Insurance. *Pediatrics.* Aug. 1999; 104(2) 195–202

Remez, Lisa. Family Planning Perspectives. Special Report: Oral Sex Among Adolescents: Is It Sex or Is It Abstinence? Nov/Dec 2000; 32(6)

Sharma, A.R., McGue, M.K., Benson, P.L. The Emotional and Behavioral Adjustment of United States Adopted Adolescents: Part II. Age at Adoption. *Children and Youth Series Review.* 1996; 18(1,2) 101–114

Stotland, N.L. Psychological Effects of Induced Abortion. *Clinical Obstetrics and Gynecology.* Sept. 1997; 40(3) 673–686

Wilf-Miron, R., Glasser, S., Sikron, F., Barell, V. Using a Health Concerns Checklist as a Bridge from Reason for Encounter to Diagnosis of Girls Attending an Adolescent Health Service. *Pediatrics.* Nov. 2000; 106(5) 1065–69

Yogman, M.W., Kindlon, D. Pediatric Opportunities with Fathers and Children. *Pediatric Annals,* Jan. 1998; 27(1) 16–22

Index